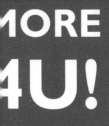
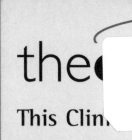 

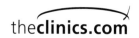

RHEUMATIC DISEASE CLINICS OF NORTH AMERICA

Mixed Connective Tissue Disease

GUEST EDITORS
Jennifer M. Grossman, MD
Daniel E. Furst, MD

August 2005 • Volume 31 • Number 3

SAUNDERS

An Imprint of Elsevier, Inc.
PHILADELPHIA   LONDON   TORONTO   MONTREAL   SYDNEY   TOKYO

W.B. SAUNDERS COMPANY
A Division of Elsevier Inc.

1600 John F. Kennedy Boulevard • Suite 1800 • Philadelphia, Pennsylvania 19103-2899

http://www.theclinics.com

RHEUMATIC DISEASE
CLINICS OF NORTH AMERICA   Volume 31, Number 3
August 2005   ISSN 0889-857X
Editor: Barton Dudlick   ISBN 1-4160-2766-1

The ideas and opinions expressed in *Rheumatic Disease Clinics of North America* do not necessarily reflect those of the Publisher. The Publisher does not assume any responsibility for any injury and/or damage to persons or property arising out of or related to any use of the material contained in this periodical. The reader is advised to check the appropriate medical literature and the product information currently provided by the manufacturer of each drug to be administered to verify the dosage, the method and duration of administration, or contraindications. It is the responsibility of the treating physician or other health care professional, relying on independent experience and knowledge of the patient, to determine drug dosages and the best treatment for the patient. Mention of any product in this issue should not be construed as endorsement by the contributors, editors, or the Publisher of the product or manufacturers' claims.

Rheumatic Disease Clinics of North America (ISSN 0889-857X) is published quarterly by Elsevier Inc. Corporate and editorial offices: 1600 John F. Kennedy Boulevard, Suite 1800, Philadelphia, PA 19103-2899. Accounting and circulation offices: 6277 Sea Harbor Drive, Orlando, FL 32887-4800. Periodicals postage paid at Orlando, FL 32862, and additional mailing offices. Subscription prices are USD 180 per year for US individuals, USD 290 per year for US institutions, USD 90 per year for US students and residents, USD 214 per year for Canadian individuals, USD 350 per year for Canadian institutions, USD 240 per year for international individuals, USD 350 per year for international institutions and USD 120 per year for Canadian and foreign students/residents. To receive student/resident rate, orders must be accompanied by name of affiliated institution, date of term, and the *signature* of program/residency coordinator on institution letterhead. Orders will be billed at individual rate until proof of status received. Foreign air speed delivery is included in all *Clinics* subscription prices. All prices are subject to change without notice. POSTMASTER: Send address changes to *Rheumatic Disease Clinics of North America*, W.B. Saunders Company, Periodicals Fulfillment, Orlando, FL 32887-4800. **Customer Service: 800-654-2452 (USA). From outside of the USA, call (+1) 407-345-4000. E-mail: hhspcs@harcourt.com.**

Reprints. For copies of 100 or more of articles in this publication, please contact the Commercial Reprints Department, Elsevier Inc., 360 Park Avenue South, New York, New York, 10010-1710; Tel.: (+1) 212-633-3813, Fax: (+1) 212-462-1935, and E-mail: reprints@elsevier.com.

Rheumatic Disease Clinics of North America is covered in *Index Medicus, Current Contents/ Clinical Medicine, Science Citation Index, ISI/BIOMED,* and *EMBASE/Excerpta Medica.*

Printed in the United States of America.

GUEST EDITORS

JENNIFER M. GROSSMAN, MD, Assistant Professor (Medicine), Division of Rheumatology, University of California at Los Angeles, Los Angeles, California

DANIEL E. FURST, MD, Carl M. Pearson Professor of Rheumatology, Division of Rheumatology, University of California at Los Angeles, Los Angeles, California

CONTRIBUTORS

EKHLAS ALHUMOUD, MD, Fellow in Allergy and Immunology, Department of Allergy and Immunology, McMaster University Medical Center, Hamilton, Ontario, Canada

MARTIN ARINGER, MD, Associate Professor, Department of Rheumatology, Internal Medicine III, Medical University of Vienna, Vienna, Austria

DAVID B. BADESCH, MD, Professor (Medicine), Division of Pulmonary Sciences and Critical Care Medicine); and Clinical Director, Pulmonary Hypertension Center, Denver, Colorado

TODD M. BULL, MD, Assistant Professor (Medicine); and Medical Director, Intensive Care Unit Anshutz Inpatient Pavillion, Division of Pulmonary Sciences and Critical Care Medicine, Pulmonary Hypertension Center, Denver, Colorado

KAREN A. FAGAN, MD, Associate Professor (Medicine), Division of Pulmonary Sciences and Critical Care Medicine, Pulmonary Hypertension Center, Denver, Colorado

THOMAS GRADER-BECK, MD, PhD, Fellow in Rheumatology, Division of Rheumatology, Johns Hopkins School of Medicine, Baltimore, Maryland

ERIC L. GREIDINGER, MD, Assistant Professor, Division of Rheumatology and Immunology, University of Miami; and Staff Physician, Miami Veterans Affairs Medical Center, Miami, Florida

JENNIFER GROSSMAN, MD, Assistant Professor (Medicine), Division of Rheumatology, University of California at Los Angeles, Los Angeles, California

STEPHEN HALL, MBBS, FRACP, Associate Professor (Medicine), Monash University, Box Hill Hospital, Melbourne, Australia

PATRICK HANRAHAN, MBBS, FRACP, Director, Goatcher Clinical Research Unit, Royal Perth Hospital, Perth, Australia

GLORIA C. HIGGINS, MD, PhD, Associate Professor (Pediatrics), Department of Pediatrics, Ohio State University, Columbus, Ohio

ROBERT W. HOFFMAN, DO, Professor and Chief, Division of Rheumatology and Immunology, University of Miami; and Chief, Rheumatology, Miami Veterans Affairs Medical Center, Miami, Florida

DAVID ISENBERG, MD, FRCP, Professor (Rheumatology), Centre for Rheumatology, University College London Hospitals, London, United Kingdom

RITA JERATH, MB, ChB, Assistant Professor (Pediatrics), Department of Pediatrics, Medical College of Georgia, Augusta, Georgia

PAUL KIM, MD, Fellow, Division of Rheumatology, University of California at Los Angeles, Los Angeles, California

RODANTHI C. KITRIDOU, MD, MACR, FACP, Professor (Medicine), Division of Rheumatology and Immunology, Department of Medicine, University of Southern California Keck School of Medicine, Los Angeles County–University of Southern California Medical Center, Los Angeles, California

INGRID E. LUNDBERG, MD, PhD, Professor (Rheumatology), Rheumatology Unit, Department of Medicine, Karolinska University Hospital, Solna, Karolinska Institute, Stockholm, Sweden

RICHARD J. MIER, MD, Director, Pediatric Services, Shriners Hospital for Children, Lexington, Kentucky

JANET E. POPE, MD, MPH, FRCPC, Director, Postgraduate Education, Division of Rheumatology; and Professor, Divisions of Rheumatology and Epidemiology and Biostatistics, Department of Medicine, Faculty of Medicine, University of Western Ontario, London, Ontario, Canada

ROBERT M. RENNEBOHM, MD, Associate Professor (Clinical Pediatrics), Department of Clinical Pediatrics, Ohio State University, Columbus, Ohio

MICHAEL SHISHOV, MD, Fellow, Division of Rheumatology, Cincinnati Children's Hospital Medical Center, Cincinnati, Ohio

JOSEF S. SMOLEN, MD, Full Professor and Head, Department of Rheumatology, Internal Medicine III, Medical University of Vienna, Vienna, Austria

GÜNTER STEINER, PhD, Associate Professor, Department of Rheumatology, Internal Medicine III, Medical University of Vienna, Vienna, Austria

JOSEPHINE SWANTON, BSc, Clinical Research Fellow, Centre for Rheumatology, University College London Hospitals, London, United Kingdom

FREDRICK M. WIGLEY, MD, Professor (Medicine), Division of Rheumatology, Johns Hopkins School of Medicine, Baltimore, Maryland

DOROTHY W. WORTMANN, MD, Clinical Associate Professor (Pediatrics), Department of Pediatrics, Oklahoma University College of Medicine, Tulsa, Oklahoma

CONTENTS

For patients who have combined features of rheumatoid arthritis, the limited cutaneous form of systemic sclerosis, and inflammatory myopathies, the concept of mixed connective tissue disease (MCTD) often helps to predict and diagnose organ problems and to educate the patient accordingly. With high titer IgG antibodies to U1 ribonucleoprotein (U1-RNP), this concept is supported by a specific serologic marker, and autoantibodies to U1-RNP and to heterogeneous nuclear ribonucleoprotein (hnRNP)-A2 display MCTD specificity with regard to the recognized epitopes. In addition, the association of MCTD with HLA-DR4 distinguishes it from systemic erythematosus lupus and systemic sclerosis, and speaks to its being a disease entity, rather than a mixture of yet undifferentiated collagen vascular diseases. The authors believe that the concept is useful in daily practice and accurate in the idea that MCTD constitutes a disease entity of its own.

Mixed connective tissue disease (MCTD) remains a controversial diagnosis. The classification criteria have changed significantly from the original description by Sharp and colleagues in 1972 after follow-up of the original and other MCTD patients. In this article we review the clinical, serologic, and genetic studies of MCTD published in the last 10 years and ask if this term is appropriate.

Pulmonary hypertension is associated with proliferative vascular abnormalities that involve small pulmonary vessels, rather than interstitial lung disease.

Mixed connective tissue disease (MCTD) is believed to be incurable and seems to have a variable prognosis. Some patients have a mild self-limited disease, whereas others develop major organ involvement that requires aggressive treatment. Because no controlled clinical trials have been performed to guide therapy in MCTD, treatment strategies must rely largely upon the conventional therapies that are used for similar problems in other rheumatic conditions (systemic lupus erythematosus, scleroderma, polymyositis). Given the heterogeneous clinical course of MCTD, therapy should be individualized to address the specific organs involved and the severity of underlying disease activity. Corticosteroids, antimalarials, methotrexate, cytotoxics (most often cyclophosphamide), and vasodilators have been used in the treatment of MCTD with varying degrees of success.

FORTHCOMING ISSUES

RECENT ISSUES

THE CLINICS ARE NOW AVAILABLE ONLINE!

Access your subscription at:
http://www.theclinics.com

ELSEVIER
SAUNDERS

Rheum Dis Clin N Am 31 (2005) xi–xii

RHEUMATIC
DISEASE CLINICS
OF NORTH AMERICA

Preface

Mixed Connective Tissue Disease

It has been an honor for us to edit this multiauthored issue of the *Rheumatic Disease Clinics of North America* on mixed connective tissue disease (MCTD). All of the authors are experts in their respective fields. The editing has been both enjoyable and educational for us. We would like to express our gratitude to the contributors for their excellent work.

In the field of medicine, the dogma is to conform to Occam's Razor, the attribution of a constellation of signs and symptoms to one diagnosis. This is certainly true in the field of rheumatology, in which careers have been made by the classification of diseases and the ability to distinguish one rheumatic illness from another. The concept of MCTD is a prime example of an effort to identify a relatively homogeneous set of patients. We feel that it is important to acknowledge up front that it has been hotly debated among rheumatologists whether or not the classification of MCTD accomplishes this goal. There are those who feel it is a worthwhile classification because it helps identify a set of patients for whom general prognostic information and perhaps more targeted diagnostic and therapeutic interventions may be provided. The arguments for the use of this classification are elegantly explored by Smolen and colleagues. Other rheumatologists have not found this classification to be useful and prefer to use the individual manifestations. Swanson and Isenberg illustrate the shortcomings of the MCTD classification and the opinion opposed to the view that MCTD is a unitary diagnosis.

With the controversy acknowledged and explored, this issue of *Rheumatic Disease Clinics of North America* then emphasizes the current state of our understanding of the pathogenesis, epidemiology, clinical manifestations, and treatment of this condition. The decision was made in the interest of space to devote added emphasis to the more protean manifestations of the disease: serologic findings, pulmonary disease, Raynaud's phenomenon, and myositis. Focus on the areas of childhood disease, disease during pregnancy, treatment, and prognosis were included because recent, readily available reviews for these topics are not available elsewhere.

0889-857X/05/$ – see front matter © 2005 Elsevier Inc. All rights reserved.
doi:10.1016/j.rdc.2005.06.001

One of the challenges of studying a rare condition is the small number of patients who have this diagnosis at any one center. The literature on MCTD is based on relatively small case series, with very few multicenter studies. We hope that one day there might be registries or multicenter cohorts established to better address the pathogenesis, diagnosis, and treatment of this condition. We will eagerly await these studies while we care for this challenging patient population.

Jennifer M. Grossman, MD
Daniel E. Furst, MD
Division of Rheumatology
University of California at Los Angeles
1000 Veterans Avenue
Box 951670, Room 32-59
Los Angeles, CA 90025-1670, USA
E-mail addresses: jgrossman@mednet.ucla.edu (J.M. Grossman)
defurst@mednet.ucla.edu (D.E. Furst)

ELSEVIER
SAUNDERS

RHEUMATIC
DISEASE CLINICS
OF NORTH AMERICA

Rheum Dis Clin N Am 31 (2005) 411–420

Does Mixed Connective Tissue Disease Exist? Yes

Martin Aringer, MD, Günter Steiner, PhD,
Josef S. Smolen, MD*

*Department of Rheumatology, Internal Medicine III, Medical University of Vienna, AKH,
Waehringer Guertel 18-20, A-1090 Vienna, Austria*

In most situations when there is a syndrome described that consists of a set of typical clinical features and is associated with a serologic marker, it is an obvious success story. This is not necessarily so in rheumatology when considering the history of mixed connective tissue disease (MCTD). Over 32 years, this concept [1] has, in some ways, split rheumatologists into two parties: some use this concept in daily clinical practice, whereas others consider it to be artificial and of little relevance.

One of the basic problems for rheumatologists is that they are still far from a complete understanding of the systemic autoimmune diseases that are encountered and treated. Thus, there often are no "diagnostic" criteria for these diseases, and the various classification criteria have been designed for scientific, rather than diagnostic, reasons. Moreover, for reasons of practicality, these criteria rely on the common organ problems or common serologic findings of the disease in question, and leave out other, less common, features of the disease in a given patient. With these limitations in mind, a lack of overlap between related disorders might trigger the question of whether another disease entity in between has been missed (Fig. 1).

Under these circumstances, the concept of MCTD would be useful if: (1) the idea of MCTD is a practical tool in clinical practice which helps to predict problems and guide the evaluation and treatment of a patient who is diagnosed with this disorder, and (2) its recognition as a distinct disease entity

* Corresponding author.
E-mail address: josef.smolen@wienkav.at (J.S. Smolen).

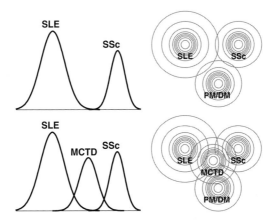

Fig. 1. If little overlap is present between two disease entities defined in a probabilistic way (by specificity and sensitivity), another disease entity likely will fit in between. DM, dermatomyositis; PM, polymyositis; SLE, systemic lupus erythematosus; SSc, systemic sclerosis.

is in concordance with the present clinical, serologic, and genetic evidence. The article attempts to evaluate and lay out the evidence for or against the existence of MCTD.

Is mixed connective tissue disease a useful concept?

There is little dispute that patients exist who present with clinical features of more than one classic rheumatic disease. In many cases, patients who have such overlap syndromes are defined as having an overlap between disease A and disease B (eg, between systemic lupus erythematosus [SLE] and rheumatoid arthritis [RA]). An occasional patient has a combination of several features, such as RA-like erosive arthritis, Raynaud's phenomenon, esophageal dysmotility and fibrosing lung disease that is typical of the limited cutaneous form of systemic sclerosis (lcSSc), an inflammatory myopathy that is reminiscent of polymyositis (PM), and SLE-like lymphocytopenia. One might call this patient's problem an RA/lcSSc/PM/SLE overlap, but will this help to explain anything? Will this be a disease entity that can be explained to the patient, taught to students, and focused on in medical science? Would not, rather, a common disease concept make life easier under such circumstances?

In some rheumatologists' experience, this patient would be likely to have high titer antinuclear antibodies (ANA) and autoantibodies against the U1 small nuclear ribonucleoprotein autoantigen (U1-snRNP), which are part of the classification criteria of MCTD [1–4]. Accordingly, this patient would be diagnosed as having MCTD and the rheumatologist may have an idea of what the disease and its therapy will be like.

Most of the criticism of the MCTD concept raises three issues: (1) the original concept of a more benign disease—which does not involve certain major organs and would respond well to low-dose corticosteroid therapy—has not turned out to be correct in follow-up investigations [5]; (2) many of the patients also satisfy criteria of a single disease entity with time [6,7]; and (3) there is not one set of widely accepted criteria for MCTD [8].

Typical disease manifestations in mixed connective tissue disease

Patients who are diagnosed as having MCTD are likely to suffer at some time from polyarthritis, myositis, Raynaud's phenomenon, puffy hands or mild sclerodactyly, interstitial lung disease, and esophageal dysmotility [2,4,9–11].

Musculoskeletal disease is common. Arthralgias or frank arthritis affect most patients who have a diagnosis of MCTD—50% to 70% are rheumatoid factor positive and about half suffer from an erosive arthritis [12–15]. Myalgias are another standard feature [1], and up to two thirds of the patients suffer from overt myositis that ranges from mild to severe [11,16]. Histologically, myositis in MCTD is indistinguishable from the myositis in patients who have PM or SLE, and immunoglobulin deposits are found in most patients [14,16].

Raynaud's phenomenon also is an important problem in MCTD [2,17–19]. Nailfold capillaroscopy of fingers demonstrated changes that were more reminiscent of SSc than SLE, but bushy formations seem to be characteristic of MCTD [20]. Moreover, in an angiographic evaluation of 13 patients who had MCTD, severe narrowing and occlusion of digital arteries were common [21].

The same kind of SSc-like intimal hyperplasia also is the pathologic correlate of the occurrence of pulmonary hypertension, which may be life-threatening [22]. In addition to pulmonary hypertension, patients who have a diagnosis of MCTD often develop interstitial lung disease; however, this usually is mild and even may go unnoticed [23]. Esophageal dysmotility and reflux disease also occur frequently in patients who have a diagnosis of MCTD, and are more similar to the situation in SSc than in SLE [24,25]. In contrast, severe renal disease is uncommon and, if present, mainly occurs in two forms: membranous glomerulonephritis (mostly) or similar to a scleroderma renal crisis [26–28].

Diseases with features similar to mixed connective tissue disease

If MCTD is not a distinct disease, but is an early stage of another disease, it is particularly important to look at these other diseases, despite our limited insight into their pathogenesis. By definition, MCTD shares features with RA, SLE, SSc, and the inflammatory muscle diseases, as well as with undifferentiated connective tissue diseases (UCTDs).

RA is a good starting point because it generally is a well-defined disease entity. RA is characterized clinically by a symmetric polyarthritis with morning stiffness; most commonly this involves joints of the hands. Although clinically apparent internal organ involvement is rare when compared with connective tissue diseases (CTDs), the arthritis is not dissimilar clinically to arthritides that are seen in CTDs, such as SLE. Although RA arthritis is erosive, lupus arthritis is not erosive in most instances, and is not associated commonly with an IgM or IgA rheumatoid factor; however, mild erosive arthritis does occur in some patients who have SLE [29,30] or other CTDs [31,32]. Likewise, some patients who have CTDs are rheumatoid factor positive [33]. It is interesting that there exists another overlap disease between RA and SSc [34]; however, this is characterized by autoantibodies that are typical of RA plus anticentromere antibodies and does not have features of other CTDs. MCTD arthritis can be erosive or nonerosive.

SLE is a complex autoimmune disease with a wide variety of autoantibodies and various organ manifestations that mostly are mediated by immune complex deposition. Raynaud's phenomenon is common [35], but normally is not associated with puffy hands or sclerodactyly. Most commonly, lupus polyarthritis is nonerosive. Myositis that is similar to MCTD myositis occurs, but is less prevalent. Esophageal involvement and interstitial lung disease are infrequent events, whereas many other organ problems can be found that normally are not seen in patients who have MCTD.

Patients who have SSc show many disease features that also are found in MCTD, and if a single connective tissue disease becomes dominant, most patients who have MCTD develop SSc [6,7]. With Raynaud's phenomenon and sclerodactyly, pulmonary hypertension, interstitial lung disease and esophageal involvement, many features are similar to those of patients who have lcSSc; however, there is little evidence of any kind of immunoglobulin deposition in SSc, and severe arthritis or myositis are less common in SSc than in MCTD. Moreover, patients who have MCTD tend to be more responsive to corticosteroids [25].

Patients who have PM, and those who have dermatomyositis (DM), in particular, often present with features other than those that are caused directly by their inflammatory myopathy (ie, Raynaud's phenomenon, arthritis, or interstitial lung disease). Their arthritis usually is nonerosive, whereas the myopathy is severe and commonly is disabling. Vascular and esophageal changes apparently stem from different pathologic processes; this suggests that MCTD is not just one form of inflammatory myopathy. Moreover, the lower third of the esophagus usually is not involved in PM/DM, as it is in MCTD.

UCTDs are defined by a limited set of clinical and serologic features that does not meet the criteria for other CTDs. Many patients who are diagnosed with MCTD present first with UCTD. In this sense, UCTDs once were seen primarily as the antechamber to differentiated CTDs. In recent years, however, the cumulative evidence suggests that most of these patients will remain in the UCTD subset [36–39]. Thus, it is not appropriate to incorporate the patients who have MCTD into the subset of those who suffer from UCTD, especially because UCTD cannot be grouped under one clinical category, whereas most patients who have MCTD fulfill the respective diagnostic criteria.

Taken together, solely on clinical grounds, there is considerable overlap between MCTD and its "related" diseases: RA, SLE, SSc, and UCTD; however, it seems to be unlikely that MCTD is just a subset of any of these mostly well-defined disease entities. Rather, some findings suggest the possibility that MCTD/SLE or MCTD/SSc overlap disease may occur.

Genetic issues

MCTD is associated with the HLA-DR4, -DR1, and (less prominently) -DR2 molecules (Table 1) [40–47]. In contrast, SLE mainly is associated with HLA-DR2 and DR3 [48,49], whereas SSc shows an association with HLA-DR5 or -DR3 [50–53] and PM/DM shows an association with HLA-DR3 [54,55]. Thus, two conclusions can be drawn: (1) there is sufficient linkage disequilibrium with certain HLA class II molecules to suggest that patients who have MCTD are not an undefined mixture who have several different disorders; and (2) the HLA-DR association that is found most frequently in MCTD is not identical to those that are found most commonly in SLE, SSc, or PM/DM—the three relevant similar diseases; therefore, it is reasonable to postulate that MCTD "fills the gap" between the others. RA has similar HLA associations, but, with the exception of erosive arthritis, it rarely shares any clinical features with MCTD, and antibodies to U1-snRNP are seen almost never in RA.

As in other CTDs, some organ manifestations are associated with specific HLA types. For example, the presence of HLA-DR3 may increase the risk of lung fibrosis in MCTD [7] and SSc [51,52,56]. Given the common occurrence of erosive arthritis in MCTD, one could argue that the shared epitope association is with the erosive arthritis itself, rather than with the disease; however, the

Table 1
HLA-DR in mixed connective tissue disease

N	Compared with	Association found	Gene/subtype	First author, year [Ref.]
24	HC	HLA-DR4/MICA4/TNF	DRB1*04, DRB1*01	Hassan, 2003 [40]
46[a]	SLE, SSc	HLA-DR4, DR2	—	Gendi, 1995 [7]
20[b]	Other CTDs	HLA-DR4	—	Hoffman, 1995 [41]
22	SLE, SSc	HLA-DR4	Dw4	Hameenkorpi, 1993 [42]
64	SLE	HLA-DR4, DR1, DR9	DRB1*0401, DRB4*0101	Dong, 1993 [43]
32	SLE	HLA-DR4	Dw4	Ruuska, 1992 [44]
27[b]	HC	HLA-DR4	DRB1*0401 (Dw4)	Kaneoka, 1992 [45]
47	HC	HLA-DR4	—	Black, 1998 [46]
35[b]	HC	HLA-DR4	—	Genth, 1987 [47]

Abbreviations: HC, matched healthy control population; MICA, MHC class I–chain-related gene A; TNF, tumor necrosis factor.

[a] Comparison with those patients developing enough features of SLE or SSc to be classified as having this CTD.

[b] DR-association with U1-snRNP antibodies.

non-RA features and the autoantibody profile remain to be explained. Taken together, the HLA evidence is in favor of MCTD as a disease that is distinct from SLE, SSc, or PM/DM, and as a disease that is T-cell dependent, given the HLA class II association.

Serologic issues

The cardinal autoantibody in MCTD is directed against the U1-snRNP (one of the major components of the spliceosome), which, in addition to the common set of Smith (Sm) core proteins, is associated specifically with the three proteins, U1-A, U1-C, and U1-70K; all of these may be targeted by U1-snRNP–specific antibodies [1,2]. The pathogenicity of U1-snRNP antibodies has not been proven, but clinical associations that were observed in patients who had SLE and SSc [57,58] might be interpreted as indicating so. U1-snRNP antibodies also are found in 20% to 30% of SLE sera, but usually at lower titers; this seems to be particularly true for the U1-70K protein [59–63].

In contrast and remarkably, antibodies to the Sm-D antigen, which also is present in the U1-snRNP (and in all other spliceosomal snRNPs), are largely pathognomonic for SLE [64,65]; patients who fulfill the criteria for MCTD rarely have autoantibodies to Sm [11]. Moreover, most patients who had UCTDs and high titer U1-snRNP antibodies fulfilled criteria for MCTD at the end of the study [66]. Antigen recognition seems to be different between SLE and MCTD. In an epitope mapping study, 94% of the patients who had MCTD, but

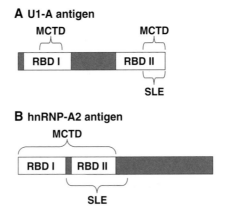

Fig. 2. Differential epitope recognition in MCTD and SLE. (*A*) Autoantibodies of patients who have MCTD recognize an epitope that is located within the RBD I of the U1-snRNP associated U1-A protein that rarely is recognized by patients who have SLE and a common epitope that is located in RBD II. (*B*) Autoantibodies from patients who have MCTD are directed specifically to a large epitope of hnRNP-A2 that contains both RBDs, whereas antibodies of patients who have SLE or RA preferentially bind to an epitope that is located within RBD II.

only 20% of the patients who had SLE, recognized the 35–58 peptide of the
U1-A protein [67]. Finally, patients who had MCTD were much less likely than
patients who had SLE to retain IgM U1-snRNP autoantibodies [68]. Therefore,
long-standing high titer IgG U1-snRNP antibodies are typical for MCTD and
convey high specificity.

In addition to differences in their immune response to U1-snRNP, patients who
have MCTD differ from patients who have SLE (and RA) in their response to
another spliceosome-associated protein, the heterogeneous nuclear RNP (hnRNP)
A2 (RA33). Antibodies against hnRNP-A2 are found in approximately one
third of patients who have either of the diseases [69–71]. The region of hnRNP-
A2 that is targeted by autoantibodies is limited to the second of the two RNA
binding domains (RBDs) in patients who have SLE and RA, whereas antibodies
of patients who have MCTD recognize a larger epitope that contains sequences
of both RBDs [11,72]. Therefore, although not pathognomonic for any of the
diseases, the antibody response against hnRNP-A2 distinguishes patients who
have MCTD from those who have SLE and RA by virtue of the difference in
epitope recognition (Fig. 2).

Summary

Taken together, there are several good, solid arguments for the existence of
MCTD as a specific disease entity. There are patients who have clinical features
that do not allow them to be grouped with patients who have SLE, lcSSc, RA, or
UCTD. These patients are likely to carry HLA-DR molecules that are not found
commonly in SLE or SSc but are associated more often with RA. They also
are likely to show a high titer autoantibody level to a largely specific portion of
the U1-snRNP protein; among patients who have UCTDs, those who have high
titer U1-snRNP antibodies usually go on to develop MCTD. Moreover, the
autoantibody response to at least one other antigen (ie, hnRNP A2), differs from
that of patients who have SLE or RA. The authors believe that the MCTD concept is a useful one that helps to diagnose, inform, and treat patients appropriately, and is well-founded on genetic and immunologic findings.

References

[1] Sharp GC, Irvin WS, Tan EM, et al. Mixed connective tissue disease—an apparently distinct
    rheumatic disease syndrome associated with a specific antibody to an extractable nuclear anti-
    gen (ENA). Am J Med 1972;52(2):148–59.
[2] Sharp GC, Irvin WS, May CM, et al. Association of antibodies to ribonucleoprotein and Sm
    antigens with mixed connective-tissue disease, systematic lupus erythematosus and other
    rheumatic diseases. N Engl J Med 1976;295(21):1149–54.
[3] Kasukawa R, Tojo T, Miyawaki S. Preliminary diagnostic criteria for classification of MCTD. In:
    Kasukawa R, Sharp GC, editors. Mixed connective tissue diseases and anti-nuclear antibodies.
    Amsterdam: Elsevier; 1987. p. 23–32.

[4] Alarcon-Segovia D, Cardiel MH. Comparison between 3 diagnostic criteria for mixed connective tissue disease. Study of 593 patients. J Rheumatol 1989;16(3):328–34.

[5] Black C, Isenberg DA. Mixed connective tissue disease–goodbye to all that. Br J Rheumatol 1992;31(10):695–700.

[6] Nimelstein SH, Brody S, McShane D, et al. Mixed connective tissue disease: a subsequent evaluation of the original 25 patients. Medicine (Baltimore) 1980;59(4):239–48.

[7] Gendi NS, Welsh KI, van Venrooij WJ, et al. HLA type as a predictor of mixed connective tissue disease differentiation. Ten-year clinical and immunogenetic followup of 46 patients. Arthritis Rheum 1995;38(2):259–66.

[8] Isenberg D, Black C. Naming names! Comment on the article by Smolen and Steiner. Arthritis Rheum 1999;42(1):191–6.

[9] Piirainen HI, Kurki PT. Clinical and serological follow-up of patients with polyarthritis, Raynaud's phenomenon, and circulating RNP antibodies. Scand J Rheumatol 1990;19(1):51–6.

[10] von Muhlen CA, Tan EM. Autoantibodies in the diagnosis of systemic rheumatic diseases. Semin Arthritis Rheum 1995;24(5):323–58.

[11] Smolen JS, Steiner G. Mixed connective tissue disease: to be or not to be? Arthritis Rheum 1998;41(5):768–77.

[12] O'Connell DJ, Bennett RM. Mixed connective tissue disease—clinical and radiological aspects of 20 cases. Br J Radiol 1977;50(597):620–5.

[13] Ramos-Niembro F, Alarcon-Segovia D, Hernandez-Ortiz J. Articular manifestations of mixed connective tissue disease. Arthritis Rheum 1979;22(1):43–51.

[14] Bennett RM, O'Connell DJ. Mixed connective tissue disease: a clinicopathologic study of 20 cases. Semin Arthritis Rheum 1980;10(1):25–51.

[15] Piirainen HI. Patients with arthritis and anti-U1-RNP antibodies: a 10-year follow-up. Br J Rheumatol 1990;29(5):345–8.

[16] Oxenhandler R, Hart M, Corman L, et al. Pathology of skeletal muscle in mixed connective tissue disease. Arthritis Rheum 1977;20(4):985–8.

[17] McHugh N, James I, Maddison P. Clinical significance of antibodies to a 68 kDa U1RNP polypeptide in connective tissue disease. J Rheumatol 1990;17(10):1320–8.

[18] Michels H. Course of mixed connective tissue disease in children. Ann Med 1997;29(5):359–64.

[19] Burdt MA, Hoffman RW, Deutscher SL, et al. Long-term outcome in mixed connective tissue disease: longitudinal clinical and serologic findings. Arthritis Rheum 1999;42(5):899–909.

[20] Granier F, Vayssairat M, Priollet P, et al. Nailfold capillary microscopy in mixed connective tissue disease. Comparison with systemic sclerosis and systemic lupus erythematosus. Arthritis Rheum 1986;29(2):189–95.

[21] Peller JS, Gabor GT, Porter JM, et al. Angiographic findings in mixed connective tissue disease. Correlation with fingernail capillary photomicroscopy and digital photoplethysmography findings. Arthritis Rheum 1985;28(7):768–74.

[22] Alpert MA, Goldberg SH, Singsen BH, et al. Cardiovascular manifestations of mixed connective tissue disease in adults. Circulation 1983;68(6):1182–93.

[23] Sullivan WD, Hurst DJ, Harmon CE, et al. A prospective evaluation emphasizing pulmonary involvement in patients with mixed connective tissue disease. Medicine (Baltimore) 1984; 63(2):92–107.

[24] Gutierrez F, Valenzuela JE, Ehresmann GR, et al. Esophageal dysfunction in patients with mixed connective tissue diseases and systemic lupus erythematosus. Dig Dis Sci 1982;27(7):592–7.

[25] Marshall JB, Kretschmar JM, Gerhardt DC, et al. Gastrointestinal manifestations of mixed connective tissue disease. Gastroenterology 1990;98(5 Pt 1):1232–8.

[26] Kobayashi S, Nagase M, Kimura M, et al. Renal involvement in mixed connective tissue disease. Report of 5 cases. Am J Nephrol 1985;5(4):282–9.

[27] Kitridou RC, Akmal M, Turkel SB, et al. Renal involvement in mixed connective tissue disease: a longitudinal clinicopathologic study. Semin Arthritis Rheum 1986;16(2):135–45.

[28] Satoh K, Imai H, Yasuda T, et al. Sclerodermatous renal crisis in a patient with mixed connective tissue disease. Am J Kidney Dis 1994;24(2):215–8.

[29] Richter CM, Steiner G, Smolen JS, et al. Erosive arthritis in systemic lupus erythematosus: analysis of a distinct clinical and serological subset. Br J Rheumatol 1998;37(4):421–4.

[30] Ostendorf B, Scherer A, Specker C, et al. Jaccoud's arthropathy in systemic lupus erythematosus: differentiation of deforming and erosive patterns by magnetic resonance imaging. Arthritis Rheum 2003;48(1):157–65.

[31] Udoff EJ, Genant HK, Kozin F, et al. Mixed connective tissue disease: the spectrum of radiographic manifestations. Radiology 1977;124(3):613–8.

[32] Baron M, Lee P, Keystone EC. The articular manifestations of progressive systemic sclerosis (scleroderma). Ann Rheum Dis 1982;41(2):147–52.

[33] Shmerling RH, Delbanco TL. The rheumatoid factor: an analysis of clinical utility. Am J Med 1991;91(5):528–34.

[34] Zimmermann C, Steiner G, Skriner K, et al. The concurrence of rheumatoid arthritis and limited systemic sclerosis: clinical and serologic characteristics of an overlap syndrome. Arthritis Rheum 1998;41(11):1938–45.

[35] Cervera R, Khamashta MA, Font J, et al. Systemic lupus erythematosus: clinical and immunologic patterns of disease expression in a cohort of 1,000 patients. The European Working Party on Systemic Lupus Erythematosus. Medicine (Baltimore) 1993;72(2):113–24.

[36] Williams HJ, Alarcon GS, Joks R, et al. Early undifferentiated connective tissue disease (CTD). VI. An inception cohort after 10 years: disease remissions and changes in diagnoses in well established and undifferentiated CTD. J Rheumatol 1999;26(4):816–25.

[37] Swaak AJ, van de Brink H, Smeenk RJ, et al. Incomplete lupus erythematosus: results of a multicentre study under the supervision of the EULAR Standing Committee on International Clinical Studies Including Therapeutic Trials (ESCISIT). Rheumatology (Oxford) 2001;40(1):89–94.

[38] Mosca M, Neri R, Bencivelli W, et al. Undifferentiated connective tissue disease: analysis of 83 patients with a minimum followup of 5 years. J Rheumatol 2002;29(11):2345–9.

[39] Bodolay E, Csiki Z, Szekanecz Z, et al. Five-year follow-up of 665 Hungarian patients with undifferentiated connective tissue disease (UCTD). Clin Exp Rheumatol 2003;21(3):313–20.

[40] Hassan AB, Nikitina-Zake L, Padyukov L, et al. MICA4/HLA-DRB1*04/TNF1 haplotype is associated with mixed connective tissue disease in Swedish patients. Hum Immunol 2003;64(2):290–6.

[41] Hoffman RW, Sharp GC, Deutscher SL. Analysis of anti-U1 RNA antibodies in patients with connective tissue disease. Association with HLA and clinical manifestations of disease. Arthritis Rheum 1995;38(12):1837–44.

[42] Hameenkorpi R, Ruuska P, Forsberg S, et al. More evidence of distinctive features of mixed connective tissue disease. Scand J Rheumatol 1993;22(2):63–8.

[43] Dong RP, Kimura A, Hashimoto H, et al. Difference in HLA-linked genetic background between mixed connective tissue disease and systemic lupus erythematosus. Tissue Antigens 1993;41(1):20–5.

[44] Ruuska P, Hameenkorpi R, Forsberg S, et al. Differences in HLA antigens between patients with mixed connective tissue disease and systemic lupus erythematosus. Ann Rheum Dis 1992;51(1):52–5.

[45] Kaneoka H, Hsu KC, Takeda Y, et al. Molecular genetic analysis of HLA-DR and HLA-DQ genes among anti-U1–70-kd autoantibody positive connective tissue disease patients. Arthritis Rheum 1992;35(1):83–94.

[46] Black CM, Maddison PJ, Welsh KI, et al. HLA and immunoglobulin allotypes in mixed connective tissue disease. Arthritis Rheum 1988;31(1):131–4.

[47] Genth E, Zarnowski H, Mierau R, et al. HLA-DR4 and Gm(1,3;5,21) are associated with U1-nRNP antibody positive connective tissue disease. Ann Rheum Dis 1987;46(3):189–96.

[48] Reinertsen JL, Klippel JH, Johnson AH, et al. B-lymphocyte alloantigens associated with systemic lupus erythematosus. N Engl J Med 1978;299(10):515–8.

[49] Scherak O, Smolen JS, Mayr WR. HLA-DRw3 and systemic lupus erythematosus. Arthritis Rheum 1980;23(8):954–7.

[50] Briggs DC, Welsh K, Pereira RS, et al. A strong association between null alleles at the C4A locus in the major histocompatibility complex and systemic sclerosis. Arthritis Rheum 1986;29(10): 1274–7.

[51] Reveille JD. Molecular genetics of systemic sclerosis. Curr Opin Rheumatol 1993;5(6):753–9.

[52] Vargas-Alarcon G, Granados J, Ibanez DK, et al. Association of HLA-DR5 (DR11) with systemic sclerosis (scleroderma) in Mexican patients. Clin Exp Rheumatol 1995;13(1):11–6.

[53] Satoh M, Akizuki M, Kuwana M, et al. Genetic and immunological differences between Japanese patients with diffuse scleroderma and limited scleroderma. J Rheumatol 1994;21(1): 111–4.

[54] Miller FW. Humoral immunity and immunogenetics in the idiopathic inflammatory myopathies. Curr Opin Rheumatol 1991;3(6):902–10.

[55] Shamim EA, Rider LG, Miller FW. Update on the genetics of the idiopathic inflammatory myopathies. Curr Opin Rheumatol 2000;12(6):482–91.

[56] Briggs DC, Vaughan RW, Welsh KI, et al. Immunogenetic prediction of pulmonary fibrosis in systemic sclerosis. Lancet 1991;338(8768):661–2.

[57] Furtado RN, Pucinelli ML, Cristo VV, et al. Scleroderma-like nailfold capillaroscopic abnormalities are associated with anti-U1-RNP antibodies and Raynaud's phenomenon in SLE patients. Lupus 2002;11(1):35–41.

[58] Asano Y, Ihn H, Yamane K, et al. The prevalence and clinical significance of anti-U1 RNA antibodies in patients with systemic sclerosis. J Invest Dermatol 2003;120(2):204–10.

[59] Mattioli M, Reichlin M. Characterization of a soluble nuclear ribonucleoprotein antigen reactive with SLE sera. J Immunol 1971;107(5):1281–90.

[60] Reichlin M, Mattioli M. Correlation of a precipitin reaction to an RNAprotein antigen and a low prevalence of nephritis in patients with systemic lupus erythematosus. N Engl J Med 1972;286(17):908–11.

[61] Habets WJ, de Rooij DJ, Hoet MH, et al. Quantitation of anti-RNP and anti-Sm antibodies in MCTD and SLE patients by immunoblotting. Clin Exp Immunol 1985;59(2):457–66.

[62] Reichlin M, van Venrooij WJ. Autoantibodies to the URNP particles: relationship to clinical diagnosis and nephritis. Clin Exp Immunol 1991;83(2):286–90.

[63] Klein Gunnewiek JM, Van De Putte LB, van Venrooij WJ. The U1 snRNP complex: an autoantigen in connective tissue diseases. An update. Clin Exp Rheumatol 1997;15(5):549–60.

[64] Tan EM, Kunkel HG. Characteristics of a soluble nuclear antigen precipitating with sera of patients with systemic lupus erythematosus. J Immunol 1966;96(3):464–71.

[65] Steiner G, Skriner K, Hassfeld W, et al. Clinical and immunological aspects of autoantibodies to RA33/hnRNP-A/B proteins–a link between RA, SLE and MCTD. Mol Biol Rep 1996; 23(3–4):167–71.

[66] Frandsen PB, Kriegbaum NJ, Ullman S, et al. Follow-up of 151 patients with high-titer U1RNP antibodies. Clin Rheumatol 1996;15(3):254–60.

[67] Barakat S, Briand JP, Abuaf N, et al. Mapping of epitopes on U1 snRNP polypeptide A with synthetic peptides and autoimmune sera. Clin Exp Immunol 1991;86(1):71–8.

[68] Vlachoyiannopoulos PG, Guialis A, Tzioufas G, et al. Predominance of IgM anti-U1RNP antibodies in patients with systemic lupus erythematosus. Br J Rheumatol 1996;35(6):534–41.

[69] Steiner G, Hartmuth K, Skriner K, et al. Purification and partial sequencing of the nuclear autoantigen RA33 shows that it is indistinguishable from the A2 protein of the heterogeneous nuclear ribonucleoprotein complex. J Clin Invest 1992;90(3):1061–6.

[70] Smolen JS, Hassfeld W, Steiner G. Anti-RA 33–a new autoantibody characteristic of rheumatoid arthritis. Isr J Med Sci 1990;26(12):693–4.

[71] Isenberg DA, Steiner G, Smolen JS. Clinical utility and serological connections of anti-RA33 antibodies in systemic lupus erythematosus. J Rheumatol 1994;21(7):1260–3.

[72] Skriner K, Sommergruber WH, Tremmel V, et al. Anti-A2/RA33 autoantibodies are directed to the RNA binding region of the A2 protein of the heterogeneous nuclear ribonucleoprotein complex. Differential epitope recognition in rheumatoid arthritis, systemic lupus erythematosus, and mixed connective tissue disease. J Clin Invest 1997;100(1):127–35.

ELSEVIER
SAUNDERS

RHEUMATIC
DISEASE CLINICS
OF NORTH AMERICA

Rheum Dis Clin N Am 31 (2005) 421–436

Mixed Connective Tissue Disease: Still Crazy After All These Years

Josephine Swanton, BSc, David Isenberg, MD, FRCP*

*Centre for Rheumatology, University College London Hospitals, Arthur Stanley House,
40-50 Tottenham Street, London W1T 4NJ, UK*

This history of most autoimmune rheumatic diseases follows a similar pattern. Astute clinicians over time recognize groups of clinical features that have a high level of association. Their careful descriptions are followed by widespread recognition, and the coining of a name ensues. Blood test abnormalities linked to these clinical features are reported, in particular the presence of one sort of autoantibody or another, and this helps to cement the idea that there are distinguishable autoimmune rheumatic diseases (ARDs). At some point an august body, such as the American College of Rheumatology (ACR), gets involved, and sets of criteria are more formally evaluated. These criteria are adjusted from time to time, but by and large diseases like rheumatoid arthritis, Sjögren's syndrome, scleroderma, myositis, and (to a lesser extent) systemic lupus erythematosus (SLE) are viewed as recognizable conditions with core sets of clinical features and serologic abnormalities.

The outstanding exception to this sort of history is a condition that continues in many rheumatologic circles to be referred to as mixed connective tissue disease (MCTD). Its history is quite different. In the early 1970s, Sharp and colleagues [1] identified through their laboratory notebooks a number of patients with high levels of antibodies to a ribonucleic protein (RNP). A review of the notes of 25 patients was claimed to have shown a number of shared clinical features, including Raynaud's phenomenon, arthralgias, mild arthritis (usually non-erosive and nondeforming), puffy hands, abnormal esophageal mobility, lymphadenopathy, and myositis. Hypergamma globulinemia occurred in 80%, and anemia and leukopenia occurred in 50%. Features more typical of lupus, such as photo-

---

* Corresponding author.
 E-mail address: d.isenberg@uch.ac.uk (D. Isenberg).

0889-857X/05/$ – see front matter © 2005 Elsevier Inc. All rights reserved.
doi:10.1016/j.rdc.2005.04.009

sensitivity, alopecia, mouth ulcers, rashes, serositis, and myocardial involvement, were said to be uncommon. Likewise, clinically apparent pulmonary, renal, and neurologic involvement was stated to be rare, vasculitis was not reported, the steroid requirement was considered low, and the outcome was considered benign with low mortality. The term MCTD was coined to capture this group of patients. Serious doubts about the existence of such a syndrome began to surface when in 1980 Nimelstein and colleagues [2] reviewed 22 out of 25 of the original patients. They expressed the following concerns about the original claims:

- Clinical evolution was observed in many patients away from inflammatory rheumatic disease toward noninflammatory scleroderma.
- A high mortality rate was noted among these patients (8 patients had died).
- The extent of association of antibodies to RNP with clinical MCTD was unclear. In particular, it was noted that not everyone with clinical MCTD had antibodies to RNP and that among Sharp's original patients some had high titers of anti-RNP antibody without displaying clear features of an overlap syndrome. They concluded that the results indicated that certain features of the patients that had originally thought to make them clinically distinct "had not held true over time."

During the next 20 years, many studies were published reporting contradictory views about the existence and nature of MCTD. Some were adamant that in the prospective follow-up of patients with overlap syndromes, the presence of high-titer, anti-RNP antibodies did not identify a particular clinical subgroup and concluded that "mixed connective tissue disease does not appear to be a distinct entity" [3] but rather an "intermediate stage in a genetically determined progression to a recognized connective tissue disease" [4]. However, patients with the antibody tended to fulfill more criteria of other diseases than those without it. A review published in 1992 put forward the view that the original definition of MCTD had changed so radically over time that the term was of little value and that it would be better to refer to patients with genuine overlapping sets of clinical features of ARDs as having undifferentiated ARD [5]. In this article, we focus on studies published in the past decade to determine whether the term MCTD (it remains entrenched in many rheumatology textbooks) is appropriate or if its use is, as Paul Simon once put it, "still crazy after all these years."

Diagnostic criteria

Four sets of diagnostic criteria have been published, those of Sharp [6], Kasukawa [7], Alarcon-Segovia [8], and Kahn [9], summarized in a review by Smolen and Steiner [10]. These four diagnostic criteria have been evaluated [11] alongside ACR criteria for other well-defined ARDs, and Alarcon-Segovia's [8] and Kahn's [9] criteria were concluded to be comparable to the highest sensitivity

(62.5% [increased to 81.3% if "myositis" is replaced with "myalgia"]) and specificity (86.3%) when tested in 45 patients with anti-RNP antibodies. When tested in-house on 593 patients with well-defined ARDs, including MCTD, SLE, scleroderma, DM/PM, and rheumatoid arthritis (RA), the sensitivity of the Alarcon-Segovia criteria rose to 100% with specificity reaching 99.6% with inclusion of serologic criteria [12]. Such high accuracies would be expected if the 80 patients who had MCTD were initially diagnosed by the same criteria. In this same study, Sharp's criteria were singled out for having a low specificity, with 11% falsely fulfilling the criteria.

Alarcon-Segovia's [8] is the simplest of the sets of criteria, involving five clinical manifestations, as opposed to 13 to 15. Requirements for diagnosis are a serologic criterion plus at least three of five clinical criteria, including synovitis or myositis. The serologic criterion is anti-RNP at a hemagglutination titre of 1:1600 or greater. The clinical criteria are (1) edema of the hands, (2) synovitis, (3) myositis, (4) Raynaud's phenomenon, and (5) acrosclerosis.

The crux of the MCTD diagnosis is the presence of high titers of antibodies to U1-RNP. In a study of 26 MCTD patients satisfying Alarcon-Segovia criteria [13], it was observed that many patients also satisfied the ACR criteria for RA or SLE, of whom many also had myositis or symptoms of systemic sclerosis (SSc). The presence of high-titer anti-RNP pushed these patients into the MCTD classification. With the serology superseding the clinical symptoms in the diagnosis, there is a risk of fitting the clinical symptoms to the antibody signs; yet, it has been suggested that the presence of these antibodies should not be essential for a diagnosis because they may not always be present throughout the clinical course. A review of Sharp's original 25 patients showed that some did not have anti-RNP antibodies despite having the classical symptoms resembling MCTD [2]. Also, the presence of anti-RNP antibodies is recognized in other ARDs. Based on these data, we believe too much weight is given to the serology at the expense of the clinical picture.

A benign disease course?

Studies have shown that MCTD is not a benign disease, and vital organs, such as the lungs, can be involved. It has a mortality rate that exceeds that of SLE, according to one report [4]. The clinical course of MCTD was observed in a retrospective study of 47 patients who fulfilled the Kasukawa criteria [7] and did not evolve into another ARD [14]. Their clinical and serologic information had been collected from presentation, diagnosis, and follow-up for more than 3 years (mean 15 years). Mean age at diagnosis was 31 years.

Table 1 summarizes the most frequent clinical features at various stages of the disease. At last follow-up, the inflammatory conditions frequently seen at diagnosis had responded to treatment (steroids or cytotoxic agents); thus, myositis, arthritis, erythematous skin rashes, swollen hands, leukopenia, serositis, Raynaud's, and esophageal hypomotility had become less frequent. As some rheu-

Table 1
Summary of the main clinical findings in a retrospective analysis of 47 patients with mixed connective tissue diseaseat various stages of disease presented in decreasing order of frequency

At presentation (74%–45%)	At diagnosis (89%–28%)	Cumulative findings (96%–43%)	At 5-y follow-up (60%–17%)
Raynaud's phenomenon	Raynaud's phenomenon	Raynaud's phenomenon	Raynaud's phenomenon
Polyarthralgia	Polyarthralgia	Polyarthralgia/ arthritis	Pulmonary dysfunction
Swollen hands	Swollen hands	Swollen hands	Sclerodactyly
—	Oesophagitis ± hypomotility	Oesophagitis ± hypomotility	Polyarthralgia/ arthritis
—	Pulmonary dysfunction	Pulmonary dysfunction	Oesophagitis ± hypomotility
—	Serositis	Erythematous skin rashes	Pulmonary hypertension
—	Sclerodactyly	Leukopaenia	Central nervous system disease
—	Erythematous skin rashes	Myositis	—
—	Leukopaenia	Sclerodactyly	—
—	Myositis	Serositis	—

Percentages represent the range of frequencies in that column.
Data from Kasukawa R, Tojo T, Miyawaki S. Preliminary diagnostic criteria for classification of mixed connective tissue disease. In: Kasukawa R, Sharp GC, editors. Mixed connective tissue diseases and antinuclear antibodies. Amsterdam: Elsevier; 1987. p. 41–7.

matologists have noted, the symptoms unresponsive to treatment (sclerodactyly, pulmonary dysfunction, and pulmonary hypertension) resemble a clinical picture of scleroderma, leading them to conclude that MCTD is a precursor of this ARD.

Sharp's original study [1] stated that clinically apparent pulmonary, renal, and neurologic disease was rare. In this study, renal disease occurred cumulatively in 11% of patients (biopsy-proven glomerulonephritis). However, at mean follow-up of 15 years, 2% had residual abnormality on biopsy. Neurologic disease occurred in 17% (this included seizures, organic brain syndrome, peripheral neuropathy, or trigeminal neuropathy) [14]. Other studies have shown that pulmonary dysfunction and esophageal hypomotility are frequently present in asymptomatic patients who have MCTD [15], and in this study both were shown to occur cumulatively in 66% by functional tests in all patients. Pulmonary dysfunction was defined by a restrictive defect on spirometry or less than 70% predicted diffusion capacity for carbon monoxide, and esophageal hypomotility was diagnosed on manometry studies. Pulmonary hypertension, diagnosed on postmortem or right heart catheter studies, was present in 23% of patients. Pulmonary hypertension was a major contributing factor to severe illness or death in 9 of the 11 patients who died in the follow-up period (two patients died of unrelated illness while their MCTD was in remission) [14]. Pulmonary hypertension was present in 6% of patients in remission, compared with 64% in the deceased group. One review reported a frequency of pulmonary involvement in MCTD as 20%–80% with interstitial pneumonitis and fibrosis in as many as 20%–65%, pleural effusion in 50%, pleurisy in 20%, and pulmonary hypertension in 10%–45% of patients who had MCTD [16].

In Burdt et al's study [14], postmortem lung specimens revealed intimal proliferation and medial hypertrophy of pulmonary arteries with little or no fibrosis. Pulmonary fibrosis has been noted to be a manifestation of MCTD in a cohort of patients that were symptomatic or had radiographic evidence of intrathoracic involvement and tends to be more severe if the predominant clinical feature is that of SSc [17]. Six out of 20 patients who had MCTD [18] with symptomatic or radiographic evidence of intrathoracic involvement died during a 6-year follow-up (diagnosis criteria: overlapping clinical features of SLE, SSc, and polymyositis; not fulfilling the criteria for other ARDs; anti-RNP–positive; anti-Sm–negative; and age over 16 years at presentation). Autopsies of three cases showed nonspecific fibrosis. Biopsies were not performed on the remaining patients, but pulmonary function tests showed a restrictive pattern in 69% of the symptomatic patients.

Description of radiographic pulmonary involvement of MCTD is similar to that of SSc and polymyositis and dermatomyositis (PM/DM). The most common abnormality is an interstitial pattern with a peripheral and basal predominance [16]. It is characterized on CT by ground-glass attenuation, septal thickening (due to infiltration of alveolar septa by lymphocytes), linear opacities, and peripheral and lower lobe predominance. Honeycombing is seen in advanced disease [19,20].

Bronchoalveolar lavage (BAL) findings of MCTD patients with radiographic evidence of interstitial lung disease [21] suggest a different inflammatory process from that in SSc or PM/DM. $CD4^+$ lymphocytes in BAL fluid were increased in MCTD compared with patients who had PM/DM, whereas CD71 positivity (found preferentially on mature tissue macrophages) was decreased in alveolar macrophages from patients who had MCTD compared with patients who had SSc, suggesting that the MCTD alveolar macrophages are less mature than those found in SSc. It was not established whether the three disease groups had comparable disease duration or duration of lung involvement. Thus, in many cases Sharp's original view of MCTD as a benign disease, with rare pulmonary, renal, and neurologic involvement, is not supported by the evidence.

A disease entity or part of autoimmune rheumatic disease evolution?

A number of studies have been undertaken to answer this question but have produced conflicting results. Selection criteria and length of follow-up differ between groups, and many patients were selected on serologic rather than clinical grounds. Furthermore, many of the studies are retrospective.

Gendi and colleagues [4], using a prospective study of patients with the greatest disease duration, concluded that only 36% of patients presenting with high titers of anti-RNP and clinical features of MCTD remained undifferentiated MCTD. The cohort of 39 patients diagnosed according to Sharp's original criteria had a mean age of 50.8 years and more than 20 years disease duration at 10-year follow-up [4]. Mean age at diagnosis was 30.7 years. The 64% differentiated into a defined ARD (11 SSc, 10 SLE, 2 RA, and 2 overlap syndromes). They concluded that MCTD is, for most patients, an intermediate stage in a genetically determined progression to a recognized connective tissue disease.

A cohort with a similar age and disease duration showed a comparable evolution rate, with only 39% of patients with anti-U1RNP antibodies retaining a diagnosis of MCTD [22]. Of 46 patients with positive anti-U1RNP antibodies who had been followed for more than 5 years with yearly serology, 13 could be classified as ARA-defined ARDs at presentation (10 SLE, two RA, and one SSc), with 33 classified as MCTD. During follow-up of these 33 patients, 18 were reclassified as SLE ($n = 5$), SSc ($n = 7$), RA ($n = 3$), or a combination of these ARD ($n = 3$). The authors concluded that the majority of patients with U1-RNP antibodies have or will develop a classified ARD within 5 years of presentation. The mean age of the patients was 49 years at study onset, mean disease duration was 17 years, and mean follow-up was 7 years. No distinction was made between patients with high or low titers of antibodies, which may have affected the frequency of diagnosis change. In these studies, Sharp's criteria were used, which have been noted to be less specific than other MCTD criteria and may have influenced the evolution rate.

By contrast, in a study of 151 patients with high-titer anti–U1-RNP antibodies [23], 26% were given a diagnosis of MCTD at presentation, and 64% had a diagnosis of MCTD by the end of the follow-up period (mean 7.1 years). The study did not state whether patients classified as having MCTD also fulfilled criteria for other ARDs or overlap syndromes, which may explain the discrepancy between the various studies. The disease duration was significantly lower than the studies mentioned previously, with 73% of the patients having disease duration of less than 2 years. The classification criteria used for diagnosis was not clearly established. Other diagnoses at presentation were SLE ($n = 11$), SSc ($n = 5$), and undifferentiated connective tissue disease (UCTD). By the end of the study, 127 patients had developed a well-defined ARD: SLE ($n = 18$), SSc ($n = 12$), and the 97 with MCTD. Therefore, only 36%–39% of patients with high titer anti-U1RNP antibodies and disease duration of more than 15 years maintain a diagnosis of MCTD, supporting the theory that MCTD is part of ARD evolution.

There is considerable overlap in terminology in the literature about UCTD and MCTD. This is further complicated by the variability in the inclusion criteria for UCTD in studies because of the lack of definitive diagnostic criteria. Selection criteria for UCTD are much less stringent than for MCTD, requiring only one or two symptoms suggestive of an ARD and a nonorgan specific autoantibody, and therefore UCTD cohorts represent a more diverse group than MCTD cohorts. Thus, symptom frequency is greater in the MCTD cohort because they have been selected for specific symptoms. Two prospective studies have been performed observing UCTD cohorts [24,25], and there are similarities in symptoms at various stages of the disease course of UCTD to those of MCTD described in a retrospective study by Burdt and colleagues [14] (Table 2). Muscle disease in the UCTD studies was rare but noted, and kidney involvement was absent. Swollen hands were noted in the Bodolay [25] study in the follow-up of the group with isolated Raynaud's phenomenon but not at presentation. Otherwise, the symptoms common to the UCTD at diagnosis and 5-year follow-up were comparable with those of MCTD. UCTD and MCTD had similar 5-year remission rates of around 20%, and the UCTD patients had a relatively high prevalence of permanent major organ damage, including erosive arthritis and lung fibrosis. The prevalence of these was not given, but both are recognized complications of MCTD [16,26]. Esophageal and pulmonary dysfunction and pulmonary hypertension were not specifically sought in the UCTD studies with functional tests, unlike in the MCTD study, and were probably underestimated. It is likely that some of the patients who had UCTD would fulfill certain criteria for MCTD, except perhaps the Alarcon-Segovia criteria [8], which requires swollen hands, myositis, or acrosclerosis for a diagnosis. It was not clear what differentiated the UCTD from MCTD, but if they follow a similar clinical course, which a comparison of this study with that of Burdt and colleagues [14] suggests, and differ only by the presence of an antibody, is differentiation valid?

To help clarify the conundrum, we have reviewed some studies of UCTD. One study compared the evolution of the well-established ARDs and UCTD [27]. Four hundred ten patients (mean age 41.5 years) identified within 12 months of ARD symptom onset, were followed for 10 years to review diagnoses and death and remission rates. One hundred ninety-seven were classified as RA, SLE, SSc, or DM/PM at baseline; 115 were classified as UCTD with at least 3 out of 11 having specific manifestations of ARD and 98 classified as a UCTD subgroup with isolated RP or undifferentiated polyarthritis. MCTD was not recognized as a defined ARD and was not discussed. A high percentage of patients was lost to follow-up over the 10 years. Diagnosis remained unchanged in the vast majority of patients with well-established ARDs, with up to 6% of the patients with SSc, RA, or SLE being given a new diagnosis by the 10-year follow-up. The patients with PM/DM had a similar evolution rate to those with UCTD, with 21% obtaining a new diagnosis (of UCTD) compared with 29% of UCTD patients (of SLE, RA, or SSc). Remission rates were similar in all groups (18% in UCTD, 15% in RA and SLE, and 21% in PM/DM) apart from SSc (no patients in remission) at 10 years. Ten-year survival was at least 87% in all diagnostic categories apart from SSc, in which it was 56%. They concluded that after 10 years, patients with well-established ARD tended to remain with the original diagnosis, and patients with UCTD tended to remain undifferentiated or to remit. The figures presented suggest a higher rate of differentiation in UCTD than in other well-defined ARDs and, excluding SSc, similar remission rates.

Other studies have looked at UCTD evolution but included MCTD as a defined ARD. One prospective study [25] recruited 665 patients with UCTD, defined in this study by the presence of at least two clinical manifestations suggestive of any ARD and at least one non-organ specific autoantibody. They

Table 2
Frequency comparison of clinical findings in studies of mixed and undifferentiated connective tissue diseases

| | MCTD | | UCTD | | | |
| | Burdt et al, 1999 [14] | | At diagnosis | | At 5 y | |
Characteristics	At diagnosis ($n = 47$)	Cumulative findings at 5 y ($n = 47$)	Danieli et al, 1999 [24] ($n = 183$)	Bodolay et al, 2003 [25] ($n = 665$)	Danieli et al, 1999 [24] ($n = 165$)	Bodolay et al, 2003 [25] ($n = 435$)
Raynaud's	89%	96%	50%	59%	52%	77%
Arthralgia/arthritis	85%	96%	37%	49%	45%	64%
Swollen hands	60%	66%	—	—		Noted, but no % given
Oesophageal dysmotility	47%[a]	66%[a]	5%[b]	—	7%[b]	—
Pulmonary dysfunction (reduced diffusion capacity)	43%[a]	66%[a]	7%[b]	—	8%[b]	—
Serositis	34%	43%	6%	10%	6%,	15%
Haematologic	30%	53%	19%	30%	24%	37%
Erythematous skin rash	30%	53%	52%	23%	52%	33%
Muscle myositis	28%	51%	0%	0.5%	0%	0.5%
Pulmonary hypertension	9%[a]	23%[a]	[b]	—	[b]	—
Sclerodermatous skin change	4%	19%	5%	—	5%	Noted, but no % given
Central and peripheral nervous systems	0%	17%	7%	9%	9%	15%
Renal	2%	11%	0%	0%	0%	0%
Sicca	Reported elsewhere as up to 1/3 of MCTD patients. Not reported here.		22%	13%	22%	15%

[a] Functional tests performed on all patients.
[b] No functional tests performed on asymptomatic patients.

Data from Setty YN, Pittman CB, Mahale AS, et al. Sicca symptoms and anti-SSA/Ro antibodies are common in mixed connective tissue disease. J Rheumatol 2002;29(3):487–9.

were followed from presentation for 5 years. Mean age was 44.3 years. Remission rate was less than 20%, and 35% evolved into a defined ARD (87 developed RA, 45 Sjögren's, 28 SLE, 26 Alarcon-Segovia criteria for MCTD, 22 vasculitis, 19 SSc, and 3 PM/DM), and 65% were said to have stable UCTD. ARD evolution was most frequent within the first 2 years of presentation (79.5%). The presence of anti–U1-RNP autoantibodies had predictive value for the evolution of MCTD along with polyarthritis in the hand joints.

A prospective, multicenter study of 165 patients with UCTD [24] with at least two clinical signs suggestive of ARD or one clinical and one serologic sign followed for 5 years showed that only 6% evolved into a defined ARD (5 SLE, 4 SS, 1 DM/PM, and 1 MCTD). Mean age was 41.5 years, and symptom onset was less than 24 months. Diagnostic criteria used for the various ARDs, including MTCD, were not clearly established.

In summary, 6%–35% of UCTD patients evolve into a well-defined ARD, and less than 20% remit during 5-year follow-up. MCTD studies discussed previously show a higher rate of evolution of over 60%, but the patients who had MCTD had longer disease duration than the patients who had UCTD who were studied much earlier in their disease course (17–20 years compared with 5–10 years). It is not clear if MCTD behaves differently from other UCTDs and therefore if it should be considered a distinct diagnosis.

Autoantibodies

Sharp [1] described MCTD around the presence of anti–U1-RNP antibodies; however, they are not diagnostic because they occur in other ARDs, including PM/DM, RA, lupus, and scleroderma. In addition, they are not always found in patients with typical MCTD symptoms. Here we summarize the nature of these antinuclear antibodies.

Eukaryotic cells contain small nuclear RNAs complexed with several proteins to make small nuclear ribonucleoproteins. The most commonly described snRNPs are U1, U2, U3, U4/6, and U5, characterized by the snRNA and a complex of a combination of proteins; A, B'/B, C, D, and 70K. They constitute a substantial part of the spliceosome, splicing premessenger RNA to functional mRNA. Their assembly is complex, requires movement to and from the nucleus, and occurs in a stepwise fashion in a specific order. The U1 RNA is complexed with three specific proteins known as 70K, A, and C and with the Sm proteins common to all the spliceosomal snRNPs. Antibodies to the Sm proteins are found predominantly in SLE and can precipitate all snRNPs. Anti–U1-RNP antibodies exclusively precipitate the U1-RNP from nuclear extracts, being directed against the proteins A, C, or 70K and in some cases the U1-RNA. Such antibodies are thought to be the hallmark for MCTD [28]. High titers are also found in SLE, SSc, and RA [23]. Many B-cell epitopes have been determined, and the major ones colocalize with the RNA binding domains of the 70K and A proteins [29]. The presence of numerous charged amino acids was also a feature in all defined antigenic sequences [30]. Some epitopes are recognized exclusively by sera from patients who have MCTD and not by sera from other patients and vice versa [10,31]. T-cell epitopes have also been described [32–34]. Autoreactive T cells specific for U1-RNP proteins have been isolated from patients with SLE and MCTD but also from healthy individuals, with no difference being found between phenotype or specificity of the T cells from these different groups [35].

A large study was performed of over 3000 patients' sera sent to a reference laboratory over 10-year period for anti-RNP testing based on undefined "clinical grounds" [36]. The sera revealed that 109 patients were initially negative but subsequently developed anti-snRNP antibodies, and another 54 patients developed a new antibody specificity to the snRNP complex. The 70k and B′/B proteins were frequent initial seroconversion targets, and A and C peptides were late targets. It was concluded that U1RNP antibodies emerged in an orderly pattern, with 70k and B′/B acting as early immunogens. This emergence may be due to spreading of the immune response to other components of U1-RNPs, as has been shown in animal models [37] when immunization with an individual U1-RNP protein or peptide results in antibodies directed against other components of the RNP, a process that requires autoreactive T cells. It has been suggested that epitope spreading plays a pathologic role in ongoing autoimmune disease [38]. Insufficient clinical information was provided to ascertain whether this process is specific to MCTD or whether it happens with all ARDs.

By contrast, in a prospective study of 29 anti-RNP–positive, diagnostically diverse patients over 65 months (disease duration about 10 years at the end of the study), individuals' antibody specificities remained constant despite the appearance of additional clinical manifestations [39], an observation supported by Margaux and colleagues [28]. The appearance or disappearance of a specificity (ie, to 70 kd, A, C, or B/B′) was rare, coinciding with disease flare and remission, respectively. Frequent symptoms noted were arthralgia, Raynaud's phenomenon, arthritis, rashes, myalgia, and sicca symptoms. High-titer, anti-RNP antibodies ($n = 18$) with multiple specificities (to 2 or 3 of the RNP peptides) were associated with Raynaud's phenomenon, puffy hands, arthritis, pulmonary fibrosis, sclerodactyly, and myositis, fulfilling the diagnostic criteria of Alarcon-Segovia for MCTD. A scarcity of serositis, nephritis, and hematologic or dermatologic manifestations was noted in these patients. Patients with low titer ($n = 7$) fit other diagnostic criteria (SLE, SS, and RA). Only 29 patients were followed, and numbers with the various combinations of specificities were small. Three patients with Raynaud's phenomenon had none of the common specificities; one had arthritis, one had puffy hands, and one had serositis. In this study, no single U1-RNP antibody specificity has been correlated with any features of MCTD, and no there was correlation between disease activity and anti-RNP titer, as has been noted in MCTD [29]. A similar lack of correlation was found in one lupus study [40]. Therefore, it was felt in these studies that U1-RNP was not a useful marker of disease activity. On the other hand, anti-U1RNA antibodies correlated with disease activity [41] in a group of patients with SLE overlap syndromes and not specifically MCTD.

In a longitudinal study of patients who had MCTD [12], autoantibodies to ENA, RNP, U1-70kd, and U1-RNA were comparable in frequency and titer in all patients in the early active phase whether or not they went on to have mild or life-threatening disease. Remission was associated with the disappearance of autoantibodies to U1-70kd and U1-RNA and a significant reduction of ENA and RNP antibodies. In the group that died, the autoantibody levels remained essentially unchanged. The presence of aCL IgG in the early active phase was significantly more frequent in the group that died than in the group that remitted.

Anti-U1RNP antibody from patients who have ARDs can directly recognize a variety of antigens on the endothelial surface of the pulmonary artery, which may be one of the triggers of endothelial cell inflammation in ARDs [42]. It was not clearly established whether this phenomenon was more likely to occur with serum from patients who have MCTD rather than other ARDs. The same group found upregulation of intercellular adhesion molecule-1, endothelial leucocyte adhesion molecule-1, and class II MHC molecules on pulmonary artery endo-thelial cells by anti–U1-RNP antibodies [43].

Other autoantibodies common to other ARDs (eg, lupus [44]) have been described in MCTD. High-titer ANA is characteristic of MCTD, but hypocom-plementemia and antibodies to double-stranded DNA are rare. SSA/Ro and SSB/ La antibodies have been demonstrated in 32.7% and 3.6% of MCTD patients, respectively, and the former was associated with malar rash and photosensitivity [27]. SSA/Ro and SSB/La antibodies were found in 55% and 14%, respectively, of 42 lupus patients but did not correlate with any clinical features in this study [41].

Anticardiolipin (aCL) antibodies are found but do not seem to be associated with clinical features of the antiphospholipid syndrome. In one study, 15% of a group of patients with MCTD ($n = 48$) had aCL antibodies, compared with 1% of healthy control subjects. No clotting events were found among the patients who had MCTD with positive aCL antibodies, whereas 26 events were documented in the SLE group with positive aCL ($n = 24/59$). This may be due to the aCL in MCTD being independent of beta-2-glycoprotein I [45,46]. aCL is associated with pulmonary hypertension with significantly higher IgG aCL titers in patients with MCTD and pulmonary hypertension than in those without the complication [47]. Anticardiolipin antibodies have been associated with pulmonary hyper-tension in lupus, and this is therefore not unique to MCTD [48].

Antibodies directed against fibrillin-1, a main component of microfibrils in the extracellular matrix of skin, are characteristic of the murine model of systemic sclerosis and are strongly associated with human diffuse systemic sclerosis. IgG antifibrillin-1 antibodies were also found to be significantly increased in frequency among patients who have MCTD ($n = 59$) or MCTD, with evidence of diffuse SSc ($n = 10$) at 34% and 30%, respectively [49]. Diagnosis for MCTD was based on overlapping features of scleroderma, myositis, or SLE with serum antibodies to U1-RNP. These features were also found in 40% of the patients who had PM/DM, which was greater than in the groups with diffuse or limited SSc (37% and 9%, respectively), limiting their specificity.

As with other ARDs, many autoantibodies are found in patients who have MCTD. Anti–U1-RNP antibodies are thought to be the hallmark of MCTD, but these are not exclusive to MCTD. Despite this, in a small study, high titers and multiple specificities of such antibodies were associated with symptoms and signs that make up the criteria for MCTD, such as puffy hands, myositis, and Raynaud's phenomenon [40]. No single specificity correlates with the clinical features, and no anti–U1-RNP antibodies seem to correlate with disease activity in MCTD [29], apart from anti–U1-RNA antibodies, which also showed some correlation in a group of SLE overlap patients [12]. The pathogenicity of anti-RNP antibodies has not been demonstrated, but early in vitro work shows antigens on pulmonary artery endothelial cells and that antigens cause upregulation of adhesion molecules.

In summary, autoantibodies seen in MCTD have some features (eg, epitopes) that are recognized exclusively by patients who have MCTD, which supports MCTD as a distinct entity, and other features (eg, the overlap of these auto-antibodies with a variety of ARDs) that do not support the validity of MCTD as a separate diagnosis.

Human leukocyte antigen association

There are variable associations between ARD and major histocompatibility complexes (MHC). RA, for example, has been strongly associated with an epitope found on DR4 subtypes DRB1*0401, 0404, 0405, and DR1 subtype DRB1*0101 [50].

A few studies have demonstrated an association with MCTD and human leukocyte antigen (HLA) DR4 [51,52]. A study comparing haplotypes of patients with SLE (fulfilling the ARA criteria) and MCTD (fulfilling the Alarcon-Segovia criteria) showed that there was a DR4 subtype, Dw4, that was found at increased frequency in 45% of patients who had MCTD compared with 18% of control subjects and 14% of patients who had SLE [53]. In this study, 52% of the patients who had MCTD had some form of DR4, compared with 28% of control subjects. An association with MICA4/HLA-DRB1*04/TNF1 haplotype was found comparing sera from 24 patients who had MCTD and 229 healthy Swedish control subjects [52]. Other studies have shown an association with HLA DR4 and the development of anti-RNP antibodies. Patients with anti–U1-RNP antibodies (with clinical RA, SLE, SSc, or MCTD) were shown to have a higher frequency of HLA DR4 allele than control subjects (66% compared with 28%). The Gm(1,3;5,21) phenotype was found in 46% of patients and in 25% of control subjects; in the patient group, the Gm(1,3;5,21) phenotype was found only in those who were DR4-positive. The DR4 and Gm(1,3;5,21) combination seemed to be related to antibody formation and not to disease expression [54].

Gendi and colleagues [4] evaluated the clinical features of the diseases and their association with HLA alleles and showed that the association with HLA DR4 was restricted to the group with arthritis. This study of 39 patients diagnosed initially with MCTD and followed for 10 years concluded that MHC antigens influence the evolution into other CTDs. Differentiation into SSc was associated with DR5. All but one of the patients who remained MCTD after 10 years were DR2 or DR4. HLA affected the disease expression, with DR1 or DR4 influencing the severity of the arthritis and DR3 being associated with keratoconjunctivitis sicca. Therefore, the association of HLA DR4 with MCTD may be a misinterpretation and may be linked to erosive arthritis rather than to the whole syndrome.

Another study found an association with HLA DR6 [55]. Comparing 28 patients' sera with antibodies to U1A or SmD1 proteins (with diagnoses of MCTD, SLE, RA, Sjögren's syndrome, and scleroderma), the DRB1*06 allele was significantly more frequent in anti-RNP–positive patients reacting with the U1A protein than in anti-RNP–positive patients not reacting to the U1A protein.

Summary

The controversy about the existence of MCTD challenges us to reflect upon the question of disease nomenclature and its utility. We identify individual diseases and give them labels as a matter of convenience and because we believe they may provide a guide to outcome and thus help us to decide what we can tell our patients about future possible complications. For patients in whom problems are straightforward (eg, an attack of measles or mumps), this approach is useful because the outcome is uniform and straightforward in most cases. However, ARDs do not fall neatly into easily distinguishable "little boxes." In addition, there are many patients who have more than one classifiable ARD. There are many patients who meet criteria for a particular disease and have a mild version of it, whereas others may die from it. Even with the ongoing refinement of classification criteria (as with SLE and RA), we must not forget that these labels are at best approximations to the underlying pathologic mechanisms, which are complex interactions of genetic, hormonal, and environmental factors. Only as these individual factors are "teased out" will we be able to accurately define individual disorders and provide accurate prognoses.

In spite of the more rigorous attempts to classify MCTD and clarification of the evolution of anti–U1-RNP antibodies, the use of the term "MCTD" remains controversial. The original description of Sharp and colleagues [1] (ie, of a benign condition with little steroid requirement always associated with high level of antibodies to nRNP and showing clear but overlapping features of other ARDs) is not tenable. Some patients have the clinical features without the antibodies, and vice versa. Some patients evolve over time from more mild overlapping ARD to more severe and more classical cases. Given the major changes in the original concept of MCTD (ie, it can no longer be considered a benign condition because pulmonary and renal disease are commonly present, a daily dose of more than 10 mg of corticosteroids is frequently required, anti-RNP antibodies are not disease specific, and clinical features of so-called "MCTD" can occur in the absence of these antibodies), it is time to move away from this controversial title. We have previously suggested "undifferentiated autoimmune rheumatic disease" as an alternative. This change would enable us to refer to another song from the Paul Simon repertoire and put "a bridge over these troubled waters."

References

[1] Sharp GC, Irvin WS, Tan EM, et al. Mixed connective tissue disease: an apparently distinct rheumatic disease syndrome associated with a specific antibody to an extractable nuclear antigen (ENA). Am J Med 1972;52:148–59.

[2] Nimelstein SH, Brody S, McSHane D, et al. Mixed connective tissue disease: a subsequent evaluation of the original 25 patients. Medicine (Baltimore) 1980;59:239–48.

[3] Lazaro MA, Maldonado Cocco JA, Catoggio LJ, et al. Clinical and serologic characteristics of patients with overlap syndrome: is mixed connective tissue disease a distinct clinical entity? Medicine 1989;68:58–65.

[4] Gendi N, Welsh K, Van Venrooij W, et al. HLA type as a predictor of mixed connective tissue disease differentiation. Arthritis Rheum 1995;38:259–66.

[5] Black C, Isenberg DA. Mixed connective tissue disease: goodbye to all that. Br J Rheumatol 1992;31:695–700.

[6] Sharp GC. Diagnostic criteria for classification of MCTD. In: Kasukawa R, Sharp GC, editors. Mixed connective tissue diseases and antinuclear antibodies. Amsterdam: Elsevier; 1987. p. 23–32.

[7] Kasukawa R, Tojo T, Miyawaki S. Preliminary diagnostic criteria for classification of mixed connective tissue disease. In: Kasukawa R, Sharp GC, editors. Mixed connective tissue diseases and antinuclear antibodies. Amsterdam: Elsevier; 1987. p. 41–7.

[8] Alarcon-Segovia D, Villareal M. Classification and diagnostic criteria for mixed connective tissue disease. In: Kasukawa R, Sharp GC, editors. Mixed connective tissue diseases and antinuclear antibodies. Amsterdam: Elsevier; 1987. p. 33–40.

[9] Kahn MF, Appeboom T. Syndrome de Sharp. In: Kahn MF, Peltier AP, Meyer O, Piette JC, editors. Les maladies systemiques. 3rd edition. Paris: Flammarion; 1991. p. 545–56.

[10] Smolen J, Steiner G. Mixed connective tissue disease: to be or not to be? Arthritis Rheum 1998;41:768–77.

[11] Amigues J, Cantagrel A, Abbal M, et al. Comparative study of 4 diagnosis criteria sets for mixed connective tissue disease in patients with anti-RNP antibodies. J Rheumatol 1996;23:2055–62.

[12] Alarcon-Segovia D, Cardiel MH. Comparison between 3 diagnostic criteria for mixed connective tissue disease: study of 593 patients. J Rheumatol 1989;16:328–34.

[13] Hassfeld W, Steiner G, Studnicka-Benke A, et al. Autoimmune response to the spliceosome: an immunologic link between rheumatoid arthritis, mixed connective tissue disease, and systemic lupus erythematosus. Arthritis Rheum 1995;38:777–85.

[14] Burdt M, Hoffman R, Deutscher S, et al. Long-term outcome in mixed connective tissue disease. Arthritis Rheum 1999;42:899–909.

[15] Sullivan WD, Hurst DJ, Harmon CE, et al. A prospective evaluation emphasising pulmonary involvement in patients with mixed connective tissue disease. Medicine (Baltimore) 1984;63:92–107.

[16] Prakash UB. Respiratory complications in mixed connective tissue disease. Clin Chest Med 1998;19:733–46.

[17] Prakash UB. Pulmonary manifestations in MCTD. Semin Respir Med 1988;9:318–24.

[18] Prakash UB. Intrathoracic manifestations in MCTD. Mayo Clin Proc 1985;60:813–21.

[19] Wiener-Kronish JP, Soinger AM, Warnock ML, et al. Severe pulmonary involvement in mixed connective tissue disease. Am Rev Respir Dis 1981;124:499–503.

[20] Prakash UBS. Lungs in mixed connective tissue disease. J Thorac Imag 1992;7:55–61.

[21] Enomoto K, Takada T, Suzuki E, et al. Bronchoalveolar lavage fluid cells in mixed connective tissue disease. Respirology 2003;8:149–56.

[22] van den Hoogen FH, Spronk PE, Boerbooms AM, et al. Longterm follow up of 46 patients with anti-(U1)snRNP antibodies. Br J Rheumatol 1994;33:1117–20.

[23] Frandsen PB, Kriegbaum NJ, Ullman S, et al. Follow up of 151 patients with high titer U1RNP antibodies. Clin Rheumatol 1996;15:254–60.

[24] Danieli M, Fraticelli P, Franceschini F, et al. Five year follow up of 165 Italian patients with undifferenitated connective tissue diseases. Clin Exp Rheumatol 1999;17:585–91.

[25] Bodolay E, Csiki Z, Szekanecz Z, et al. Five year follow-up of 665 Hungarian patients with undifferentiated connective tissue disease (UCTD). Clin Exp Rheumatol 2003;21:313–20.

[26] O'Connell DJ, Bennett RM. Mixed connective tissue disease: clinical and radiological aspects of 20 cases. Br J Rheumatol 1977;50:620–5.

[27] Williams HJ, Alarcon GS, Joks R, et al. Early undifferentiated connective tissue disease (CTD): VI. An inception cohort after 10 years: disease remissions and changes in diagnoses in well established and undifferentiated CTD. J Rheumatol 1999;26:816–25.

[28] Margaux J, Haymen G, Palazzo E, et al. Clinical usefulness of antibodies to U1snRNP proteins in MCTD and SLE. Rev Rheum Engl Ed 1998;65:378–86.

[29] Klein Gunnewiek JMT, Van Venrooij WJ. Autoantigens contained in the U1 small nuclear ribonucleoprotein complex. In: Van Venrooij WJ, Maini RN, editors. Manual of biological disease markers. Dordrecht: Kluwer Academic Publishers; 1994. p. B3.1.

[30] Gunnewiek J, Van De Putte L, Van Venrooij W. The U1snRNP complex: an autoantigen in connective tissue diseases: an update. Clin Exp Rheumatol 1997;15:549–60.

[31] Skiner K, Sommergruber WH, Tremmel V, et al. Anti A2/RA33 autoantibodies are directed to the RNA-binding region of the A2 protein of the heterogeneous nuclear ribonucleoprotein complex. J Clin Invest 1997;100:127–35.

[32] O'Brien RM, Cram DS, Coppel RL, et al. T-cell epitopes on the 70kDa protein of the U1 RNP complex in autoimmune rheumatologic disorders. J Autoimmun 1990;3:747–57.

[33] Okkubo M, Yamamoto K, Kato T, et al. Detection and epitope analysis of autoantigen-reactive T cells to the U1 small nuclear ribonucleoprotein A protein in autoimmune disease patients. Arthritis Rheum 1995;38:1170–2.

[34] Fenning S, Wolff-vorbeck G, Hackl W, et al. T cell lines recognizing the 70 kDa protein of the U1 snRNP. Clin Exp Immunol 1995;101:408–13.

[35] Hoffman RW, Takeda Y, Sharp GC, et al. Human T cell clones reactive against UsnRNP autoantigens from connective tissue disease patients and healthy individuals. J Immunol 1993;151:6460–9.

[36] Greidinger EL, Hoffman RW. The appearance of U1RNP antibody specificities in sequential autoimmune human antisera follows a characteristic order that implicates the U1-70kd and B'/B proteins as predominant U1 RNP immunogens. Arthritis Rheum 2001;44:368–75.

[37] Craft J, Peng S, Fuji T, et al. Autoreactive T cells in murine lupus: origins and roles in autoantibody production. Immunol Res 1999;19:245–57.

[38] Vanderlugt CL, Miller SD. Epitope spreading in immune-mediated diseases: implications for immunotherapy. Nat Rev Immunol 2002;2:85–95.

[39] Lundberg I, Nyman U, Pettersson I, et al. Clinical manifestations and anti U1snRNP antibodies: a prospective study of 29 anti-RNP antibody positive patients. Br J Rheumatol 1992;31:811–7.

[40] Isenberg DA, Garton M, Reichlin MW, et al. Long-term follow-up of autoantibody profiles in black female lupus patients and clinical comparison with Caucasian and Asian patients. Br J Rheumatol 1997;36:229–33.

[41] Hoet RM, Koornneef I, de Rooij DJ, et al. Changes in anti-U1RNA antibody levels correlate with disease activity in patients with systemic lupus erythematous overlap syndrome. Arthritis Rheum 1992;35:1202–10.

[42] Okawa-Takatsuji M, Aotsuka S, Uwatoko S, et al. Endothelial cell-binding activity of anti U1 ribonucleoprotein antibodies in patients with connective tissue diseases. Clin Exp Immunol 2001;126:345–54.

[43] Okawa-Takatsuji M, Aotsuka S, Fujinami M, et al. Up regulation of intercellular adhesion molecule-1 (ICAM-1), endothelial leucocyte adhesion molecule-1 (ELAM-1) and class II MHC molecules in pulmonary artery endothelial cells by antibodies against U1RNP. Clin Exp Immunol 2001;126:345–54.

[44] Moss KE, Ioannou Y, Sultan SM, et al. Outcome of a cohort of 300 patients with systemic lupus erythematosus attending a dedicated clinic for over two decades. Ann Rheum Dis 2002;61:409–13.

[45] Komatireddy GR, Wang GS, Sharp GC, et al. Antiphospholipid antibodies among anti-U1 70kD autoantibody positive mixed connective tissue disease patients. J Rheumatol 1997;24: 319–22.

[46] Menoca LLF, Amengual O, Atsumi T, et al. Most anticardiolipin antibodies in mixed connective tissue disease are beta glycoprotein independent. J Rheumatol 1998;25:190–1.

[47] Nishimaki T, Aotsuka S, Kondo H, et al. Immunological analysis of pulmonary hypertension in connective tissue diseases. J Rheumatol 1999;26:2357–62.

[48] Asherson RA, Mackworth-Young CG, Boey ML, et al. Pulmonary hypertension in systemic lupus erythematosus. BMJ 1983;287:1024–5.

[49] Tan FK, Arnett FC, Antohi S, et al. Autoantibodies to the extracellular matrix microfibrillar protein fibrillin1 in patients with scleroderma and other connective tissue diseases. J Immunol 1999;13:1066–72.

[50] Watanabe Y, Tokunaga K, Matsuki K, et al. Putative amino acid sequence of HLA-DRB chain contributing to RA susceptibility. J Exp Med 1989;169:2263–8.

[51] Black CM, Maddison PJ, Welsh KI, et al. HLA and immunoglobulin allotypes in mixed connective tissue disease. Arthritis Rheum 1988;31:131–4.

[52] Hassan A, Nikitina-Zake L, Padyukov L, et al. MICA4/JLA-DRB1*04/TNF1 haplotype is associated wit mixed connective tissue disease in Swedish patients. Hum Immunol 2003;64: 290–6.

[53] Ruuska P, Hameenkorpi R, Forsberg S, et al. Differences in HLA antigens between patients with mixed connective tissue disease and systemic lupus erythematosus. Ann Rheum Dis 1992;51:52–5.

[54] Genth E, Zarnowski H, Mierau R, et al. HLA-DR4 and Gm(1,3;5,21) are associated with U1-nRNP antibody positive connective tissue disease. Ann Rheum Dis 1987;46:189–96.

[55] Dumortier H, Abbal M, Fort M, et al. MHC class II gene associations with autoantibodies to U1A and SmD1 proteins. Int Immunol 1999;11:249–57.

RHEUMATIC
DISEASE CLINICS
OF NORTH AMERICA

ELSEVIER
SAUNDERS

Rheum Dis Clin N Am 31 (2005) 437–450

Autoantibodies in the Pathogenesis of Mixed Connective Tissue Disease

Eric L. Greidinger, MD[a,b], Robert W. Hoffman, DO[a,b],*

[a]Division of Rheumatology and Immunology, University of Miami, Miami, FL, USA
[b]Miami Veterans Affairs Medical Center, Miami, FL, USA

As it is defined currently, to have mixed connective tissue disease (MCTD) is to have an autoantibody-producing process. To meet any of the four widely used classification criteria for a diagnosis of MCTD, patients are required to have anti-ribonucleoprotein (RNP) autoantibodies [1]. Since MCTD was described initially by Sharp and colleagues [2], the nature of the autoantibody response in MCTD has become better understood regarding what autoantibodies develop in MCTD, when autoantibodies develop in MCTD, what components of the immune system are needed to develop autoantibodies in MCTD, and whether autoantibodies can indicate prognosis in MCTD. Knowledge has emphasized the importance of autoantibodies in MCTD, and pointed out that humoral immunity alone is insufficient to account for MCTD pathogenesis. In addition to B cells and their products, data (for review see [3]) strongly support the concept that T cells and other immune system constituents play key roles in disease pathogenesis. This information has led to new hypotheses on the pathogenesis of MCTD that integrate features of the autoantibody response with issues in autoantigen recognition, T-cell activation, and stimulation of innate immunity.

This work was supported by the Department of Veterans Affairs and by National Institutes of Health Grants AR 43308 and AR 48055.

* Corresponding author. Division of Rheumatology and Immunology, University of Miami, Dominion Towers, Room 602 (D4-10), 1400 NW 10th Avenue, Miami, FL 33136.

  E-mail address: RHoffman@med.miami.edu (R.W. Hoffman).

Types of autoantibodies in mixed connective tissue disease

As in other rheumatic autoimmune syndromes, the autoantibodies that are present in MCTD prominently include immunoglobulin class-switched to IgG [4], with variable region mutations selecting for high affinity for their autoantigen targets [5]. These features, along with the presence of apparent antigen spreading to multiple structurally unrelated autoantigens on the same macromolecule, have led to the inference that the autoimmune responses in MCTD largely are antigen driven [6,7]. Further supporting this view are recent observations that antibodies that are specific for structures formed when multiple elements of the U1-RNP interact also can be identified in patients who have MCTD [8], and that immunization with epitopes on the surface of the U1-RNP complex are more capable than masked epitopes of inducing experimental autoimmune disease [9].

The specificities of autoantibodies that are relevant to MCTD include antibodies that fulfill diagnostic criteria for MCTD, other autoantibodies that are seen frequently in patients who have MCTD, and autoantibodies that suggest alternative diagnoses in RNP-positive patients. U1-RNP is the target of autoantibodies that fulfill classification criteria for anti-RNP antibodies in MCTD. This nuclear macromolecule complex plays an essential role in the splicing of pre-mRNA into mRNA. The U1-RNP is composed of an RNA backbone, the U1-RNA, three proteins that are highly specific to the U1-RNP (the U1-A, U1-C, and U1-70kD proteins), plus a series of additional proteins that is common to multiple U-RNP- and RNA-splicing macromolecules (Fig. 1). The U1-associated

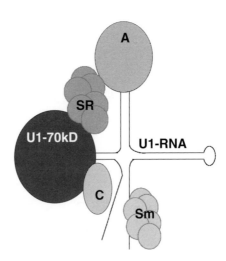

Fig. 1. The U1-RNP. The U1-RNA has double-stranded secondary structure. The U1-70kD protein binds specifically to the first stem-loop; the U1-A protein binds similarly to the second stem-loop. The Sm proteins bind to an area on a fourth stem-loop (not pictured). The SR and U1-C proteins participate in protein–protein interactions with other members of the U1-RNA.

proteins that are not specific to the U1-RNP include the Sm (Smith) proteins and a series of splicing factors that is rich in serine and arginine residues (SR proteins).

A complete understanding of the immune response to U1-RNP antigens is complicated by the fact that the protein components of U1-RNA are susceptible to a variety of posttranslational modifications as part of their catalytic function (eg, glycosylation, phosphorylation) and as a response to stress stimuli (eg, apoptotic cleavage, oxidative fragmentation, isoaspartyl formation). Patients who have established disease typically have autoantibodies to multiple U1-RNP–associated structures [7,10]. Antibodies that recognize the modified and the unmodified forms of RNP antigens exist [11]. Modified autoantigens were shown to be potentially more immunogenic than unmodified forms in animal models [12].

Although anti–U1-RNP antibodies are part of the diagnostic criteria for MCTD, this does not imply that they necessarily play any role in the development of the disease. There are two major potential roles that U1-RNP antibodies could play in MCTD that are considered further later in this article: (1) whether U1-RNP antigens are relevant for breaking tolerance and driving the autoimmune response that seems to be at the heart of the MCTD, and (2) whether immune responses to U1-RNP autoantigens mediate the forms of tissue injury that are observed in MCTD.

Although they do not complex with U1-RNP strongly or closely mimic the structure of U1-RNP, several non–U1-RNP antigens also are frequent targets of autoimmunity in patients who have MCTD. This includes other protein autoantigens, such as heterogeneous nuclear ribonucleoprotein (hnRNP) A2 and Ro/(Sjögren's syndrome antigen A) SS-A [13,14]; nucleotides, such as TS1-RNA [15]; and phospholipid moieties [16]. In animal models that were immunized extrinsically against individual RNPs, immune responses diversified to other MCTD-associated autoantigens [17,18]; this suggests that pathways of antigen spreading may exist between these structures. Like U1-RNP, the other autoantigen targets in MCTD often can be modified structurally in apoptosis [19,20]. Moreover, many of the non–U1-RNP antigens that are targeted in MCTD also are RNPs; this is consistent with the idea that protein–nucleic acid complexes are targeted preferentially in systemic autoimmunity [21]. Several hypotheses have been offered to account for putative preferential autoimmunity to RNPs in MCTD. These include the potential for structural homology/molecular mimicry between antigen targets, and conventional antigen spreading to targets that colocalize in the same macromolecule. Other explanations are under consideration, including the hypothesis that patients who have MCTD preferentially develop autoantibodies to a wide variety of apoptotically modified RNA binding proteins as a result of: (1) an inability to clear potentially proinflammatory macromolecules efficiently through noninflammatory pathways [22]; (2) incomplete baseline B- and T-cell tolerance to apoptotically modified antigen forms [23], and (3) the innate immunity-stimulating effects that are conferred on such complexes by their RNAs [24]. Alternatively, one might hypothesize that T cells that are reactive against an initial autoantigen might have degeneracy in their antigen specificity that predictably leads to coreactivity against a subset of these other antigen targets [25].

Groups of patients have been described that develop a rheumatic disease overlap syndrome that is similar to MCTD, but who do not have autoantibodies to U1-RNP. In at least some of these cases, autoantibodies to non-U1-RNP autoantigens that are seen frequently in MCTD can be found [26]. These observations demonstrate, at a minimum, that U1-RNP autoimmunity is not necessary for the development of a rheumatic overlap syndrome. It also is possible that some of these cases reflect the same underlying disease process as classic MCTD, only in a host with immunogenetic or developmentally induced resistance to U1-RNP autoimmunity. Furthermore, one could speculate that this group of antigens, rather than U1-RNP antigens, might be critical pathogenic triggers to the development of the autoimmune response, the induction of tissue injury, or both, even in classic MCTD.

Although U1-RNP antibodies are part of the classification criteria for MCTD, these antibodies are not specific for MCTD. Patients who have other diagnoses or no diagnosis also have these antibodies [7]. The other diagnoses that are associated with U1-RNP positivity include alternate connective tissue diseases (CTDs), such as systemic lupus erythematosus (SLE) or scleroderma. Some additional autoantibodies that are highly specific for a non-MCTD diagnosis, such as double-stranded DNA (dsDNA) in SLE or topoisomerase I in scleroderma, are infrequent in MCTD and may suggest an alternative diagnosis. In our experience, high titers of Sm antibodies, particularly Sm-D, are highly suggestive of SLE and are uncommon in MCTD. We (unpublished observations, 2005) and others [27,28] observed that Sm-D antibodies that are specific for the folded form of the protein are a strong risk factor for the development of lupus nephritis. Certain viral infections also may induce antibodies that cross-react with components of the U1-RNP, notably Epstein-Barr virus in the case of the Sm-B antigen and cytomegalovirus in the case of U1-70kD [29,30]. A patient who presents with additional antibodies that suggest acute infection with one of these organisms actually may be less likely to have MCTD than clinical illness because of their viral infection. It is rare for normal humans who have recovered from acute viral infection to maintain persistently detectable titers of these antibodies [31]. Conversely, a distant history of exposure to a molecular mimic infectious agent may play a role in the development of anti-RNP autoimmunity in patients who have CTD [32].

Timing of the autoantibody response in mixed connective tissue disease

By looking at banked serum samples of military recruits who later were diagnosed with SLE, James and colleagues [32,33] observed that many autoantibodies precede the development of clinical symptoms of rheumatic disease by years. Two notable exceptions were antibodies to dsDNA, and antibodies to

RNP, both of which typically developed within 1 year of a clinical diagnosis. Although the cohort of patients that was studied by James and colleagues was diagnosed with lupus, patients that met classification criteria for MCTD were not excluded; this suggests that this same pattern of RNP antibodies developing proximate to the onset of clinical disease also is likely to exist in MCTD. Just as a subset of dsDNA antibodies was shown to be able to mediate autoimmune tissue injury directly [34], an implication of these results is that a subset of RNP antibodies also may be similarly pathogenic.

Among RNP autoantibodies, the order in which RNP proteins are targeted in humans also has been defined further [7]. Most typically, antibodies to U1-70kD develop first, and are followed by antibodies to the Sm-B protein. Successive spreading of the immune response includes the U1-A and U1-C proteins, followed by Sm-D. It must be emphasized, however, that nearly half of all patients who have anti-RNP may have alternative patterns of antibody development and spread. Within the anti–U1-70kD response, we observed several patients who had antibodies to the apoptotically modified form of the protein at high titer, before substantial titers of antibodies to the native form of U1-70kD are found [35]. Conversely, we have yet to identify patients who have MCTD with antibodies to the native form of 70k who also do not have antiapoptotic 70k antibodies. This suggests that the apoptotic form of U1-70kD may be the antigen toward which U1-RNP tolerance is first broken in many patients who have MCTD [11]. Thus, the idea that an apoptotically modified autoantigen may drive the development of autoimmunity is a common theme between MCTD immunopathogenesis and models of lupus immunopathogenesis [36,37].

The order of evolution of antibodies in the New Zealand Black/White (NZB/W) F1 model of lupus—a system that is susceptible to anti-RNP responses—differs from that seen in humans. In the NZB/W animals, initial responses most typically develop against the U1-A protein, a peptide that is not known to be susceptible to posttranslational modification in apoptosis [38]. Analysis of these mice also reveals that autoantibodies to non–U1-RNP DNA and RNA binding proteins often develop concurrently with, or precede, the onset of anti–U1-RNP responses [39]. This suggests that hyperreactivity to nucleic acid binding proteins may play a more profound role in the immune responses in NZB/W animals than in humans who have MCTD, such that a posttranslationally modified autoantigen form (apoptotic 70k) is not required to break tolerance in the autoimmunity-susceptible mouse, but may be required in humans. When we immunize human HLA-DR4 transgenic mice with an epitope of the apoptotic form of U1-70kD, antibodies to 70k develop first, and are followed by the apparently simultaneous spreading of the immune response to other U1-RNP proteins and to non-U1 autoantigens [35]. In contrast, immunization with alternative peptides from 70k are less likely to induce anti-70k immunity, and have not been observed to lead to spreading. Thus, nonautoimmune prone mice seem to have similar requirements as humans for the induction of anti-RNP autoimmunity, and may represent a fruitful model for further discovery regarding MCTD immunopathogenesis.

Prerequisites for autoantibody induction in mixed connective tissue disease

Given that all autoantibodies are secreted by B cells, a functional B-cell compartment is necessary for the development of autoantibodies. Anti-RNP antibodies are among the specificities that can be identified from specialized B-cell subsets (such as B1 B cells and marginal zone B cells) that spontaneously produce "natural antibodies" in normal hosts [40]; however, B cells alone do not seem to be able to induce significant titers of MCTD autoantibodies or clinical disease autonomously. Rather, there is a strong correlation between the B-cell responses and T-cell responses to MCTD autoantigens [41]. T cells seem to be critical for the development and propagation of significant anti-RNP antibody responses [42]. Adoptive transfer of anti-RNP reactive T cells was sufficient to induce anti-RNP autoantibodies in susceptible mice [43]. Anti–U1-RNP T-cell responses, in turn, are linked to HLA-DR4 [44], and are (presumably) dependent on the presence of appropriate antigen-presenting cells in a permissive state of activation. The clinical expression of MCTD and anti-70k antibodies also have been linked to HLA-DR4 [45,46]. These results suggest that although autoantibodies are used clinically to define anti-RNP autoimmunity, a critical step in the development of anti-RNP autoimmunity occurs at the T-cell level. Moreover, it implies that antigen-presenting cells that are capable of inducing the kind of T-cell response that is observed in MCTD also must be a prerequisite for inducing pathogenic MCTD autoimmunity (see Ref. [3] for review of autoantigen-reactive human T cells and pathogenesis). A requirement for the coexistence of B cells and non-B cell antigen-presenting cells for the stimulation of anti-RNP T cells was observed in an animal model of spontaneous autoimmunity [47].

In the absence of highly penetrant genetically determined spontaneous autoimmunity, additional costimulatory signals are needed to induce proimmune antigen presentation to autoreactive T cells. An intercurrent infectious process could provide the necessary stimulus to induce antigen-presenting cells that are primed to provide proinflammatory signals. Alternatively, the ability of U1-RNA to act as an endogenous adjuvant for the development of a proinflammatory state—by way of activation of toll-like receptor (TLR)-3 signaling—also may play a role in this process [24]. U1-RNA also might induce innate immunity through other cellular RNA sensors, including TLRs 7 and 8 and protein kinase R [48,49]. After anti-RNP autoantibodies develop, the ability of RNA-containing immune complexes to induce proinflammatory responses, including type I interferon secretion from dendritic cell populations, also is likely to amplify these effects [50].

Anti-RNP T cells that are cloned from patients tend to be CD4 Th0 cells [3]. These cells are restricted in their antigen targeting to a small set of epitopes that is recognized by a spectrum of T-cell receptors of remarkably limited diversity within individual patients over time, and between patients [44]; however, these cells are able to support the production of multiple structurally diverse autoantibodies that are found in patients who have MCTD [51].

Even after tolerance is broken at the B-cell level and significant titers of IgG anti-RNP autoantibodies appear, production of these autoantibodies does not persist indefinitely. A substantial fraction of patients that is diagnosed clinically with MCTD eventually enters a long-lasting disease remission. Such remissions seem to be preceded by progressive shrinkage of the diversity of autoantibodies, and, ultimately, in the disappearance of anti-RNP antibodies [32]. The factors that allow some patients to extinguish their autoimmune response over time, whereas other patients confront implacably persistent or even progressive auto-immune responses, have not been defined conclusively. The extent of differentiation of pathogenic autoantibody-secreting cells into T cell–autonomous long-lived plasma cells could be a factor in determining the susceptibility of MCTD to remission in a given patient [52].

One additional aspect of the autoantibody spectrum that is observed in MCTD is that it tends not to include disease-associated autoantibodies that are connected with other rheumatic diagnoses. It may be that some patients who are diagnosed with other rheumatic diseases do have features of MCTD, but are diagnosed with a different condition because the clinical manifestations they have are dominated by features that are atypical for MCTD (eg, dsDNA antibodies and lupus glomerulonephritis). Thus, one also could argue that an additional prerequisite for the development of MCTD autoantibodies is the absence of additional lesions in the control of autoimmune responses that would permit an alternative, more broadly targeted autoimmune process to develop. For example, one could hypothesize that MCTD is distinguished from lupus by a susceptibility to autoimmune responses to apoptotically modified RNP complexes, rather than a more general susceptibility to immunity to apoptotically modified structures [53]. In this regard, it is of interest that some of the mediators that lead to clearance of apoptotic material and amelioration of autoimmunity (eg, C-reactive protein) seem to be efficient in binding to RNPs [54,55], whereas other pathways of apoptotic clearance whose deficiencies have been associated with increased risk of SLE are not known to have this specificity [56–58].

Autoantibodies and prognosis in mixed connective tissue disease

Ultimately, the ability to predict prognosis in MCTD based on autoantibody profiling will depend on whether MCTD autoantibodies mediate amplification of the autoimmune response itself, or development of MCTD-associated tissue injury. In either case, serially identifying and quantitating pathogenic antibodies will have immediate relevance to the management of the disease; however, if the experience with dsDNA antibodies in lupus is a guide, truly pathogenic auto-antibodies may be a small and hard-to-distinguish subset of a larger group of autoantibodies with similar specificities [59]. If autoantibodies are not directly pathogenic, measuring them is likely to be, at best, somewhat predictive of the likely clinical course and manifestations for a population of patients, but of questionable predictive value for individual patients.

Two lines of evidence suggest that anti-RNP antibodies do mediate tissue injury. Firstly, cutaneous neonatal lupus erythematosus was reported in a child who was born to a mother who had MCTD in whom RNP antibodies, but not Ro/SS-A or La/SS-B antibodies, were present [60]. The neonatal lupus syndrome is believed to occur as a result of transplacental carriage of maternal autoreactive IgG, in a local tissue context that is conducive to the development of injury [61]. Secondly, a small literature is developing that associates anti-RNP antibodies with organ-specific tissue targets that are consistent with those attacked in clinical MCTD. In addition to apoptotic RNP particles proposed to be present in sun-exposed skin [62], this also includes reactivity between RNP antibodies and the respiratory tract, another major target of MCTD manifestations [63]. Because passive transfer of MCTD autoantibodies has not been correlated with induction of lung lesions (or with several other aspects of the MCTD clinical phenotype), it is likely that nonhumoral immune mechanisms also play important roles in MCTD manifestations. The association of lung disease in MCTD with a distinct HLA-DR haplotype [64], and the enhancement in HLA-DR$^+$/CD4$^+$ T cells in bronchoalveolar lavage fluid of patients who have CTD lung disease argues for a direct pathogenic role of T cells in MCTD lung disease [65]. The recent development of an animal model of MCTD-like interstitial lung disease after immunization with an RNP peptide may lead to a better understanding of these issues [34].

This mouse model of induced anti-RNP autoimmunity also provides some evidence that the anti-RNP immune response itself can induce the amplification of autoimmunity against other structures. Animals that were immunized with an epitope of apoptotically modified U1-70kD developed a diversifying autoimmune response, whereas mice that were immunized under identical conditions with control antigens did not. This diversifying immune response includes IgG antibodies to epitopes on endogenous U1-70kD that were not part of the immunogen; antibodies to other U1-RNP proteins; and antibodies to non-U1-RNP autoantigens, including at least one human autoantigen that is recognized in its apoptotically modified; but not its intact; form [34].

Until further research is done, data on the prognostic value of autoantibodies in MCTD are limited. An initial challenge in this area is the absence of validated clinical indices to measure disease activity in MCTD. To the extent that this issue can be addressed, titers of anti-RNP antibodies have not been associated with disease activity [66]. Although one study suggested that changes in titers of U1-RNA antibodies are correlated with lupus-like manifestations of disease activity [67], assays for U1-RNA themselves are poorly standardized and of limited availability to clinicians in most areas; this makes this observation primarily one of research relevance. Although the observation of epitope shrinkage preceding clinical remission was made on a large MCTD cohort [51], this has not been validated prospectively as a predictor of subsequent remission.

Some of the non–U1-RNP autoantibodies that occur in MCTD have been reported to have diagnostic or prognostic significance in other disease processes. Antibodies to Ro have been associated with Sjögren's syndrome, cutaneous lupus, and neonatal lupus [68,69]. Antibodies to hnRNP A2 have been associated with rheumatoid arthritis (RA) and lupus [70]. Antibodies to phospholipids have been associated with a syndrome of thrombosis, pregnancy loss, and thrombocytopenia [71]. Variability exists in how predictive these antibodies are of similar manifestations in MCTD. Antiphospholipid antibodies that are found in MCTD are less likely to be associated with these manifestations than antiphospholipid antibodies in lupus [72]. Antibodies to β-2 gycoprotein-1 are less common in patients who have MCTD and antiphospholipid antibodies than in lupus [73]. Anti-Ro in MCTD is associated with subacute cutaneous lupus-like cutaneous disease, but not with keratoconjunctivitis sicca [14]. The situation with hnRNP A2 antibodies in MCTD has been studied in particular detail and may be instructive to other antigen systems. Human B-cell epitope mapping studies by Skriner and colleagues [70] showed that the antisera of patients who had lupus or RA target an epitope in the second RNA binding domain of the molecule. Sera of patients who have MCTD do not recognize this epitope, but do recognize a conformational epitope that is composed of most of the first and second RNA-binding domains. Patients who have lupus, but not patients who have MCTD and anti-hnRNP immunity, have a high prevalence of RA-like erosive arthropathy [74]; this suggests that the differential targeting of MCTD sera versus RA and lupus sera may be clinically relevant. The variable prognostic significance of these non–U1-RNP antibodies in MCTD in comparison with other autoimmune syndromes leads to the following conclusions: (1) the fact that patients who have MCTD can target different areas of these autoantigens suggests that details of the mechanisms that mediate autoimmunity are likely to differ between MCTD and other rheumatic diseases; (2) in many respects, MCTD seems to behave as a distinct syndrome, and generalizations that are drawn from data from these other diseases may not apply to MCTD [75]; and (3) currently available data, albeit incomplete, are more compelling for the theory that U1-RNP antibodies mediate tissue injury in MCTD.

A unified model for autoantibodies in mixed connective tissue disease

Based on the evidence that was articulated above, we construct the following model of RNP autoantibodies in MCTD pathophysiology: a physiologic stressor, such as a viral infection or UV light exposure, induces high quantities of apoptotic material (Fig. 2). In a host with a defect in the clearance of RNP-containing apoptotic particles, these particles encounter circulating immunoglobulin and dendritic cells. U1-RNA and similar endogenous RNA adjuvants induce dendritic cell activation and antigen presentation by way of TLR signaling, and potentially augmented by local Fc receptor ligation [76]. In a host with a compatible MHC haplotype, these cells induce activation of U1-70kD and other autoantigen-specific circulating T cells that have escaped central tolerization by deletion in the thymus. At a concurrent or subsequent physiologic stressor that leads to a shower of apoptotic material, B cells that have escaped

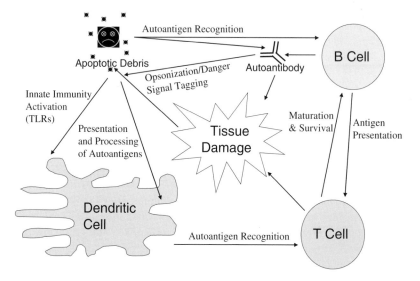

Fig. 2. A model of MCTD pathogenesis. Constituents of dead cells (apoptotic debris) that fail to be cleared through noninflammatory pathways provide proinflammatory innate immune signals (including through TLRs), and are recognized by autoantibodies. This activates B cells and opsonizes the dead cell material for more efficient uptake and presentation by antigen-presenting cells (potentially including dendritic cells and B cells themselves). Through antigen-specific signals with MHC-bound autoantigen and nonspecific proinflammatory second signals, T cells become activated, resist apoptosis, and mature into memory and effector cells. These, in turn, produce proinflammatory mediators, induce differentiation and maturation of B cells, and directly mediate cell injury. B cells under these influences avoid apoptosis and produce high quantities of avid, complement-fixing antibodies that induce tissue injury at sites of autoantigen recognition.

anergy or deletion by being specific for apoptotically modified RNA-binding proteins, including U1-70kD, are exposed to their cognate antigen in a proimmune context (potentially as a result of direct TLR recognition on B-1 and marginal zone B cells or to the effects on conventional B cells of dendritic cells and T-cell upregulation of surface costimulatory molecules plus cytokine release); this leads to maturation into IgG-secreting activated B cells. These B cells continue to be activated and secrete autoantibodies as long as they have access to antigen and to tonic costimulation. In a subset of such subjects, the autoantibodies (and antigen-specific T cells) that are produced are capable of mediating tissue injury and lead to the presentation of a rheumatic syndrome. In other individuals, previous infection with an Epstein-Barr–like virus induces a degree of B-cell hyperreactivity—and through molecular mimicry—leads to an anti–Sm-B T-cell and B-cell response. In conjunction with the autoimmunity against apoptotic U1-70kD and other structures that developed as above, this anti–Sm-B response is permissive of broader diversification of the autoimmune response, to include immunity to a wide range of U1-RNP and other MCTD-associated antigens. The resultant autoimmune response and autoantibodies are capable of mediating the features of tissue injury that are expressed in full-blown MCTD. In a subset of patients, the factors that lead to tonic activation of T and B cells supporting the autoreactive response eventually abate, and epitope shrinkage and disease remission ensue. To the extent that disease-induced tissue injury leads to additional physiologic stress and release of apoptotic material, untreated active disease will have a tendency to auto-amplify in intensity.

References

[1] Amigues JM, Cantagrel A, Abbal M, et al. Comparative study of 4 diagnosis criteria sets for mixed connective tissue disease in patients with anti-RNP antibodies. Autoimmunity Group of the Hospitals of Toulouse. J Rheumatol 1996;23(12):2055–62.
[2] Sharp GC, Irvin WS, Tan EM, et al. Mixed connective tissue disease—an apparently distinct rheumatic disease syndrome associated with a specific antibody to an extractable nuclear antigen (ENA). Am J Med 1972;52:148–59.
[3] Hoffman RW. T cells in the pathogenesis of systemic lupus erythematosus. Clin Immunol 2004; 113(1):4–13.
[4] Vlachoyiannopoulos PG, Guialis A, Tzioufas G, et al. Predominance of IgM anti-U1RNP antibodies in patients with systemic lupus erythematosus. Br J Rheumatol 1996;35(6):534–41.
[5] de Wildt RM, Ruytenbeek R, van Venrooij WJ, et al. Heavy chain CDR3 optimization of a germline encoded recombinant antibody fragment predisposed to bind the U1A protein. Protein Eng 1997;10(7):835–41.
[6] Fatenejad S, Bennett M, Moslehi J, et al. Influence of antigen organization on the development of lupus autoantibodies. Arthritis Rheum 1998;41(4):603–12.
[7] Greidinger EL, Hoffman RW. The appearance of U1 RNP antibody specificities in sequential autoimmune human antisera follows a characteristic order that implicates the U1–70 kd and B′/B proteins as predominant U1 RNP immunogens. Arthritis Rheum 2001;44(2): 368–75.
[8] Murakami A, Kojima K, Ohya K, et al. A new conformational epitope generated by the binding of recombinant 70-kd protein and U1 RNA to anti-U1 RNP autoantibodies in sera from patients with mixed connective tissue disease. Arthritis Rheum 2002;46(12):3273–82.
[9] McClain MT, Lutz CS, Kaufman KM, et al. Structural availability influences the capacity of autoantigenic epitopes to induce a widespread lupus-like autoimmune response. Proc Natl Acad Sci USA 2004;101(10):3551–6.
[10] Utz PJ, Hottelet M, van Venrooij WJ, et al. Association of phosphorylated serine/arginine (SR) splicing factors with the U1-small ribonucleoprotein (snRNP) autoantigen complex accompanies apoptotic cell death. J Exp Med 1998;187(4):547–60.
[11] Greidinger EL, Foecking MF, Ranatunga S, et al. Apoptotic U1–70 kd is antigenically distinct from the intact form of the U1–70-kd molecule. Arthritis Rheum 2002;46(5):1264–9.
[12] Mamula MJ, Gee RJ, Elliott JI, et al. Isoaspartyl post-translational modification triggers autoimmune responses to self-proteins. J Biol Chem 1999;274(32):22321–7.
[13] Skriner K, Sommergruber WH, Tremmel V, et al. Anti-A2/RA33 autoantibodies are directed to the RNA binding region of the A2 protein of the heterogeneous nuclear ribonucleoprotein complex. Differential epitope recognition in rheumatoid arthritis, systemic lupus erythematosus, and mixed connective tissue disease. J Clin Invest 1997;100(1):127–35.
[14] Setty YN, Pittman CB, Mahale AS, et al. Sicca symptoms and anti-SSA/Ro antibodies are common in mixed connective tissue disease. J Rheumatol 2002;29(3):487–9.
[15] Ikeda K, Takasaki Y, Hirokawa K, et al. Clinical significance of antibodies to TS1-RNA in patients with mixed connective tissue disease. J Rheumatol 2003;30(5):998–1005.

[16] Komatireddy GR, Wang GS, Sharp GC, et al. Antiphospholipid antibodies among anti-U1–70 kDa autoantibody positive patients with mixed connective tissue disease. J Rheumatol 1997; 24(2):319–22.

[17] Deshmukh US, Lewis JE, Gaskin F, et al. Immune responses to Ro60 and its peptides in mice. I. The nature of the immunogen and endogenous autoantigen determine the specificities of the induced autoantibodies. J Exp Med 1999;189(3):531–40.

[18] Steiner G, Shovman O, Skriner K, et al. Induction of anti-RA33 hnRNP autoantibodies and transient spread to U1-A snRNP complex of spliceosome by idiotypic manipulation with anti-RA33 antibody preparation in mice. Clin Exp Rheumatol 2002;20(4):517–24.

[19] Thiede B, Dimmler C, Siejak F, et al. Predominant identification of RNA-binding proteins in Fas-induced apoptosis by proteome analysis. J Biol Chem 2001;276(28):26044–50.

[20] Rutjes SA, van der Heijden A, Utz PJ, et al. Rapid nucleolytic degradation of the small cytoplasmic Y RNAs during apoptosis. J Biol Chem 1999;274(35):24799–807.

[21] Tan EM. Antinuclear antibodies: diagnostic markers and clues to the basis of systemic auto-immunity. Pediatr Infect Dis J 1988;7(5 Suppl):S3–9.

[22] Rosen A, Casciola-Rosen L. Clearing the way to mechanisms of autoimmunity. Nat Med 2001; 7(6):664–5.

[23] Casciola-Rosen L, Andrade F, Ulanet D, et al. Cleavage by granzyme B is strongly predictive of autoantigen status: implications for initiation of autoimmunity. J Exp Med 1999;190(6):815–26.

[24] Hoffman RW, Gazitt T, Foecking MF, et al. U1 RNA induces innate immunity signaling. Arthritis Rheum 2004;50(9):2891–6.

[25] De Silva-Udawatta M, Kumar SR, Greidinger EL, et al. Cloned human TCR from patients with autoimmune disease can respond to two structurally distinct autoantigens. J Immunol 2004; 172(6):3940–7.

[26] Zimmermann C, Steiner G, Skriner K, et al. The concurrence of rheumatoid arthritis and limited systemic sclerosis: clinical and serologic characteristics of an overlap syndrome. Arthritis Rheum 1998;41(11):1938–45.

[27] Riemekasten G, Marell J, Trebeljahr G, et al. A novel epitope on the C-terminus of SmD1 is recognized by the majority of sera from patients with systemic lupus erythematosus. J Clin Invest 1998;102(4):754–63.

[28] Burdt MA, Hoffman RW, Deutscher SL, et al. Long-term outcome in mixed connective tissue disease: longitudinal clinical and serologic findings. Arthritis Rheum 1999;42(5):899–909.

[29] McClain MT, Rapp EC, Harley JB, et al. Infectious mononucleosis patients temporarily recognize a unique, cross-reactive epitope of Epstein-Barr virus nuclear antigen-1. J Med Virol 2003;70(2):253–7.

[30] Newkirk MM, van Venrooij WJ, Marshall GS. Autoimmune response to U1 small nuclear ribonucleoprotein (U1 snRNP) associated with cytomegalovirus infection. Arthritis Res 2001; 3(4):253–8.

[31] Marshall BC, McPherson RA, Greidinger E, et al. Lack of autoantibody production associated with cytomegalovirus infection. Arthritis Res 2002;4(5):R6.

[32] James JA, Neas BR, Moser KL, et al. Systemic lupus erythematosus in adults is associated with previous Epstein-Barr virus exposure. Arthritis Rheum 2001;44(5):1122–6.

[33] Arbuckle MR, McClain MT, Rubertone MV, et al. Development of autoantibodies before the clinical onset of systemic lupus erythematosus. N Engl J Med 2003;349(16):1526–33.

[34] Mason LJ, Ravirajan CT, Rahman A, et al. Is alpha-actinin a target for pathogenic anti-DNA antibodies in lupus nephritis? Arthritis Rheum 2004;50(3):866–70.

[35] Greidinger EL, Foecking MF, Magee J, et al. A major B cell epitope present on the apoptotic but not the intact form of the U1–70-kDa ribonucleoprotein autoantigen. J Immunol 2004; 172(1):709–16.

[36] Baumann I, Kolowos W, Voll RE, et al. Impaired uptake of apoptotic cells into tingible body macrophages in germinal centers of patients with systemic lupus erythematosus. Arthritis Rheum 2002;46(1):191–201.

[37] Potter PK, Cortes-Hernandez J, Quartier P, et al. Lupus-prone mice have an abnormal response to thioglycolate and an impaired clearance of apoptotic cells. J Immunol 2003;170(6):3223–32.

[38] Laderach D, Koutouzov S, Bach JF, et al. Concomitant early appearance of anti-ribonucleo-protein and anti-nucleosome antibodies in lupus prone mice. J Autoimmun 2003;20(2):161–70.

[39] Monneaux F, Dumortier H, Steiner G, et al. Murine models of systemic lupus erythematosus: B and T cell responses to spliceosomal ribonucleoproteins in MRL/Fas(lpr) and (NZB x NZW) F(1) lupus mice. Int Immunol 2001;13(9):1155–63.

[40] Okawa-Takatsuji M, Aotsuka S, Uwatoko S, et al. The B cell repertoire in patients with sys-temic autoimmune diseases: analysis of Epstein-Barr virus (EBV)-inducible circulating precur-sors that produce autoantibodies against nuclear ribonucleoprotein (nRNP). Clin Exp Immunol 1992;90(3):415–21.

[41] Holyst MM, Hill DL, Hoch SO, et al. Analysis of human T cell and B cell responses against U small nuclear ribonucleoprotein 70-kd, B, and D polypeptides among patients with sys-temic lupus erythematosus and mixed connective tissue disease. Arthritis Rheum 1997;40(8): 1493–503.

[42] Yan J, Mamula MJ. Autoreactive T cells revealed in the normal repertoire: escape from nega-tive selection and peripheral tolerance. J Immunol 2002;168(7):3188–94.

[43] Keech CL, Farris AD, Beroukas D, et al. Cognate T cell help is sufficient to trigger anti-nuclear autoantibodies in naive mice. J Immunol 2001;166(9):5826–34.

[44] Greidinger EL, Foecking MF, Schafermeyer KR, et al. T cell immunity in connective tissue disease patients targets the RNA binding domain of the U1–70kDa small nuclear ribonucleo-protein. J Immunol 2002;169(6):3429–37.

[45] Hoffman RW, Sharp GC, Deutscher SL. Analysis of anti-U1 RNA antibodies in patients with connective tissue disease. Association with HLA and clinical manifestations of disease. Arthritis Rheum 1995;38(12):1837–44.

[46] Hoffman RW, Rettenmaier LJ, Takeda Y, et al. Human autoantibodies against the 70-kd polypeptide of U1 small nuclear RNP are associated with HLA-DR4 among connective tissue disease patients. Arthritis Rheum 1990;33(5):666–73.

[47] Monneaux F, Briand JP, Muller S. B and T cell immune response to small nuclear ribo-nucleoprotein particles in lupus mice: autoreactive CD4(+) T cells recognize a T cell epitope located within the RNP80 motif of the 70K protein. Eur J Immunol 2000;30(8):2191–200.

[48] Heil F, Hemmi H, Hochrein H, et al. Species-specific recognition of single-stranded RNA via toll-like receptor 7 and 8. Science 2004;303(5663):1526–9.

[49] Balachandran S, Roberts PC, Brown LE, et al. Essential role for the dsRNA-dependent pro-tein kinase PKR in innate immunity to viral infection. Immunity 2000;13(1):129–41.

[50] Lovgren T, Eloranta ML, Bave U, et al. Induction of interferon-alpha production in plasmacytoid dendritic cells by immune complexes containing nucleic acid released by necrotic or late apoptotic cells and lupus IgG. Arthritis Rheum 2004;50(6):1861–72.

[51] Greidinger EL, Gazitt T, Jaimes KF, et al. Human T cell clones specific for heterogeneous nuclear ribonucleoprotein A2 autoantigen from connective tissue disease patients assist in autoantibody production. Arthritis Rheum 2004;50(7):2216–22.

[52] Hoyer BF, Moser K, Hauser AE, et al. Short-lived plasmablasts and long-lived plasma cells con-tribute to chronic humoral autoimmunity in NZB/W mice. J Exp Med 2004;199(11):1577–84.

[53] Greidinger EL. Apoptosis in lupus pathogenesis. Front Biosci 2001;6:D1392–402.

[54] Szalai AJ, Weaver CT, McCrory MA, et al. Delayed lupus onset in (NZB x NZW)F1 mice expressing a human C-reactive protein transgene. Arthritis Rheum 2003;48(6):1602–11.

[55] Du Clos TW. C-reactive protein reacts with the U1 small nuclear ribonucleoprotein. J Immunol 1989;143(8):2553–9.

[56] Navratil JS, Watkins SC, Wisnieski JJ, et al. The globular heads of C1q specifically recognize surface blebs of apoptotic vascular endothelial cells. J Immunol 2001;166(5):3231–9.

[57] Cohen PL, Caricchio R, Abraham V, et al. Delayed apoptotic cell clearance and lupus-like autoimmunity in mice lacking the c-mer membrane tyrosine kinase. J Exp Med 2002;196(1): 135–40.

[58] Bickerstaff MC, Botto M, Hutchinson WL, et al. Serum amyloid P component controls chromatin degradation and prevents antinuclear autoimmunity. Nat Med 1999;5(6):694–7.

[59] Alarcon-Segovia D, Tumlin JA, Furie RA, et al. LJP 394 Investigator Consortium. LJP 394 for

the prevention of renal flare in patients with systemic lupus erythematosus: results from a randomized, double-blind, placebo-controlled study. Arthritis Rheum 2003;48(2):442–54.

[60] Fujiwaki T, Urashima R, Urushidani Y, et al. Neonatal lupus erythematosus associated with maternal mixed connective tissue disease. Pediatr Int 2003;45(2):210–3.

[61] Buyon JP, Clancy RM. Neonatal lupus syndromes. Curr Opin Rheumatol 2003;15(5):535–41.

[62] Greidinger EL, Casciola-Rosen L, Morris SM, et al. Autoantibody recognition of distinctly modified forms of the U1–70-kd antigen is associated with different clinical disease manifestations. Arthritis Rheum 2000;43(4):881–8.

[63] Okawa-Takatsuji M, Aotsuka S, Uwatoko S, et al. Increase of cytokine production by pulmonary artery endothelial cells induced by supernatants from monocytes stimulated with autoantibodies against U1-ribonucleoprotein. Clin Exp Rheumatol 1999;17(6):705–12.

[64] Gendi NS, Welsh KI, Van Venrooij WJ, et al. HLA type as a predictor of mixed connective tissue disease differentiation. Ten-year clinical and immunogenetic followup of 46 patients. Arthritis Rheum 1995;38(2):259–66.

[65] Suzuki E, Tsukada H, Ishida T, et al. Correlation between the numbers of gammadelta T cells and CD4$^+$ HLA-DR$^+$ T cells in broncho-alveolar lavage fluid from patients with diffuse lung disease. Tohoku J Exp Med 2002;196(4):231–40.

[66] Margaux J, Hayem G, Palazzo E, et al. Clinical usefulness of antibodies to U1snRNP proteins in mixed connective tissue disease and systemic lupus erythematosus. Rev Rhum Engl Ed 1998;65(6):378–86.

[67] Hoet RM, Koornneef I, de Rooij DJ, et al. Changes in anti-U1 RNA antibody levels correlate with disease activity in patients with systemic lupus erythematosus overlap syndrome. Arthritis Rheum 1992;35(10):1202–10.

[68] Simmons-O'Brien E, Chen S, Watson R, et al. One hundred anti-Ro (SS-A) antibody positive patients: a 10-year follow-up. Medicine (Baltimore) 1995;74(3):109–30.

[69] Sonesson SE, Salomonsson S, Jacobsson LA, et al. Signs of first-degree heart block occur in one-third of fetuses of pregnant women with anti-SSA/Ro 52-kd antibodies. Arthritis Rheum 2004;50(4):1253–61.

[70] Skriner K, Sommergruber WH, Tremmel V, et al. Anti-A2/RA33 autoantibodies are directed to the RNA binding region of the A2 protein of the heterogeneous nuclear ribonucleoprotein complex. Differential epitope recognition in rheumatoid arthritis, systemic lupus erythematosus, and mixed connective tissue disease. J Clin Invest 1997;100(1):127–35.

[71] Cervera R, Piette JC, Font J, et al. Euro-Phospholipid Project Group. Antiphospholipid syndrome: clinical and immunologic manifestations and patterns of disease expression in a cohort of 1,000 patients. Arthritis Rheum 2002;46(4):1019–27.

[72] Komatireddy GR, Wang GS, Sharp GC, et al. Antiphospholipid antibodies among anti-U1–70 kDa autoantibody positive patients with mixed connective tissue disease. J Rheumatol 1997; 24(2):319–22.

[73] Mendonca LL, Amengual O, Atsumi T, et al. Most anticardiolipin antibodies in mixed connective tissue disease are beta2-glycoprotein independent. J Rheumatol 1998;25(1):189–90.

[74] Richter Cohen M, Steiner G, Smolen JS, et al. Erosive arthritis in systemic lupus erythematosus: analysis of a distinct clinical and serological subset. Br J Rheumatol 1998;37(4):421–4.

[75] Smolen JS, Steiner G. Mixed connective tissue disease: to be or not to be? Arthritis Rheum 1998;41(5):768–77.

[76] Boule MW, Broughton C, Mackay F, et al. Toll-like receptor 9-dependent and -independent dendritic cell activation by chromatin-immunoglobulin G complexes. J Exp Med 2004;199(12): 1631–40.

RHEUMATIC
DISEASE CLINICS
OF NORTH AMERICA

Rheum Dis Clin N Am 31 (2005) 451–464

ELSEVIER
SAUNDERS

Pulmonary Vascular Manifestations of Mixed Connective Tissue Disease

Todd M. Bull, MD*, Karen A. Fagan, MD,
David B. Badesch, MD

Division of Pulmonary Sciences and Critical Care Medicine, Pulmonary Hypertension Center, University of Colorado School of Medicine, 4200 East Ninth Avenue, Box C-272, Denver, CO 80262, USA

Mixed connective tissue disease (MCTD) refers to a disease process with combined clinical features characteristic of systemic lupus erythematous (SLE), scleroderma, and polymyositis-dermatomyositis (PM/DM) [1]. The characteristic laboratory abnormalities in patients who have MCTD include high-titer (> 1:1000), speckled, antinuclear antibodies (ANAs); high levels of antibody against RNAse-sensitive extractable nuclear antigen; and the presence of auto-antibodies against uridienerich snRNP. The three disease processes with which MCTD shares clinical characteristics (SLE, scleroderma, and PM/DM) are associated with pulmonary pathology. MCTD is also associated with distinct clinical and pathologic pulmonary manifestations (Box 1). This article focuses on the pulmonary vasculature manifestations of MCTD. We briefly discuss associations between MCTD and interstitial lung disease, pleural disease, and alveolar hemorrhage.

The pulmonary vasculature

Pulmonary circulation is a high-capacitance, low-resistance system able to accommodate significant increases in cardiac output with little increase in pulmonary artery (PA) pressure. Through the recruitment of closed vessels and the distension of previously opened vasculature, pulmonary circulation can ac-

---

* Corresponding author.
E-mail address: Todd.Bull@UCHSC.edu (T.M. Bull).

0889-857X/05/$ – see front matter © 2005 Elsevier Inc. All rights reserved.
doi:10.1016/j.rdc.2005.04.010   *rheumatic.theclinics.com*

Box 1. Respiratory diseases associated with mixed connective
tissue disease

- Pulmonary hypertension
- Interstitial lung disease
- Pleural effusion
- Alveolar hemorrhage
- Diaphragmatic dysfunction
- Aspiration pneumonitis/pneumonia
- Thromboembolic disease
- Obstructive airways disease
- Pulmonary infections
- Pulmonary vasculitis

commodate a fourfold increase in flow with relatively small increases in PA pressure. The lung vasculature normally accepts the entire blood output from the right ventricle, and, although the blood flow to the lungs is greater than the flow to any other organ, normal mean pulmonary arterial pressure remains less then one sixth of mean systemic arterial pressure.

Increases in PA pressure can be caused by passive and active changes or by structural remodeling. Passive changes refer to alterations in pulmonary pressure not associated with vessel contraction. These alterations include increases or decreases in blood viscosity, changes in the volume of blood crossing the pulmonary vasculature, and back pressure from left-sided cardiac and valvular dysfunction. Active changes refer to contraction or relaxation of vascular smooth muscle in response to neurogenic, humoral, or chemical stimuli. Hypoxia is an example of a potent chemical stimulus that results in vasoconstriction. Humoral substances that affect the pulmonary circulation include the endogenous vasoconstrictor endothelin and the endogenous vasodilators prostacyclin and nitric oxide. Structural remodeling refers to changes in the cellular composition of the pulmonary vascular bed. These changes include intimal hypertrophy, smooth muscle cell proliferation, endothelial cell proliferation, and the formation of plexiform lesions. These pathologic changes are discussed in greater detail below.

Pulmonary arterial hypertension

Clinically, pulmonary arterial hypertension (PAH) is defined as a mean pulmonary artery pressure of greater than 25 mm Hg at rest and greater than 30 mm Hg with exercise in patients with a normal pulmonary capillary wedge pressure. Patients who have PAH commonly present with the insidious onset of dyspnea on exertion. The diagnosis is often delayed because more common causes of dyspnea are considered first. Fatigue is another common manifestation of PAH, and frequently patients and clinicians initially attribute this symptom to deconditioning. Later manifestations of pulmonary hypertension include findings consistent with right ventricular dysfunction, such as lower extremity edema and ascites. The predominant sight of pathology in patients who have PAH is the precapillary pulmonary vasculature. Histologically, the precapillary vessels in patients who have PAH develop increased wall thickness, distal extension of smooth muscle, the formation of a neointima, and an abnormal proliferation of endothelial cells resulting in the characteristic pathologic lesion of PAH, the plexiform lesion (Fig. 1). A diverse and well-defined array of diseases is associated with these same pathologic changes within the pulmonary vasculature and clinically in severe PAH (Box 2). It is difficult to differentiate between these diseases by histologic examination of the pulmonary vasculature alone.

When an underlying etiology of PAH cannot be detected, the condition is referred to as "IPAH" (previously "primary pulmonary hypertension"). IPAH is a rare disease with an incidence of only one to two cases per million people in the general population [2]. Severe pulmonary hypertension occurring in association with another disease process, such as connective tissue disease (CTD), is more common. Many investigators believe that IPAH may be associated with an unrecognized underlying autoimmune disease process. Evidence supporting this possibility includes a high incidence of ANAs in patients with IPAH and association with autoimmune thyroiditis and increased incidence of certain MHC molecules in patients who have IPAH [3–7].

PAH occurring in association with CTD is pathologically similar to other forms of severe pulmonary hypertension [8]. The etiology of PAH in patients who have CTD is unknown. Cool and colleagues [9] reported the presence of inflammatory cells surrounding the plexiform lesions in patients who had PAH

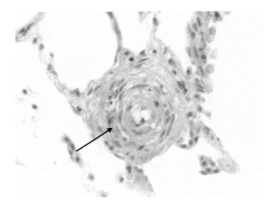

Fig. 1. Plexiform lesion from a patient diagnosed with MCTD and PAH. The plexiform lesion (*arrow*) is a characteristic pathologic finding in this disease process.

Box 2. Clinical classification of pulmonary arterial hypertension

- Idiopathic (IPAH)
- Familial (FPAH)
- Associated with (APAH)
- Collagen vascular disease
- Congenital systemic-to-pulmonary shunts
- Portal hypertension
- HIV-1 infection
- Drugs and toxins
- Other: thyroid disorders, glycogen storage disease, Gaucher disease, hereditary hemorrhagic telangiectasia, hemoglobino-pathies, myeloproliferative disorders, splenectomy

---

related to CREST syndrome, possibly indicating an inflammatory mechanism. Quismorio and colleagues [10] found antinuclear antibody and rheumatoid factor within the cells of the pulmonary vasculature in two patients who had PAH related to SLE. Others have reported IgG and complement fraction deposits in the vascular endothelium of patients who had SLE [11–13]. In some cases, pulmonary hypertension developing in patients with an underlying CTD can be attributed to pulmonary parenchymal disease, such as interstitial lung disease. The parenchymal destruction results in hypoxia and thus pulmonary vasoconstriction. Thromboembolic disease due to an underlying hypercoaguable state associated with some forms of CTD can also result in pulmonary hypertension. However, these abnormalities do not explain the vascular remodeling and severe pressure elevation typical of most cases of PAH associated with CTD.

Raynaud's phenomenon is commonly reported in patients who have scleroderma, SLE, and MCTD. The presence of pulmonary hypertension in patients who have SLE and CREST syndrome with Raynaud's phenomenon is common [13–15]. The perceived association between Raynaud's phenomenon and PAH has led to the "pulmonary Raynaud's" hypothesis in which pulmonary arterial vasospasm is believed to contribute to the development of pulmonary hypertension [16,17]. This hypothesis remains unproven.

HIV-1 and human herpesvirus-8 have been associated with IPAH [18–21]. The mechanisms by which these viral infections might cause PAH remain unclear. Viral infection has not been associated with the development of PAH in patients who have CTD.

Germline mutations in bone morphogenic protein receptor II (BMPRII) are associated with familial and sporadic forms of IPAH [22–24]. The mechanisms by which these mutations could contribute to the development of pulmonary hypertension are unclear. There is not a recognized association between mutations in BMPRII and PAH related to CTD [25,26].

Mixed connective tissue disease and pulmonary arterial hypertension

Severe pulmonary hypertension (Fig. 2) is a potentially devastating manifestation of MCTD, associated with high morbidity and mortality. Esther and colleagues [27] performed a prospective evaluation of pulmonary function in 26 patients who had MCTD. Twenty of the 26 patients had a decreased diffusing capacity on pulmonary function tests. Nine of the patients underwent right heart catheterization, and seven were diagnosed with PAH. Weiner-Kronish and colleagues [28] reported on a series of five patients with MCTD and pulmonary pathology. Three of the five patients had severe pulmonary hypertension. Autopsy series have demonstrated medial hypertrophy, intimal proliferation, and plexiform lesions, as have been observed in scleroderma-associated pulmonary hypertension and IPAH [29].

Treatment of pulmonary arterial hypertension associated with connective tissue disease

There have been no trials specifically addressing the therapy of MCTD-associated PAH. A number of studies investigating the treatment of pulmonary hypertension have included patients who had PAH associated with MCTD or the "scleroderma spectrum of disease." Therapy for PAH includes anticoagulation, oxygen, diuretics, and pulmonary vascular vasodilators. We restrict our discussion to the use of FDA-approved medications for the treatment of PAH with a brief discussion of potential future therapeutic options. We also discuss the

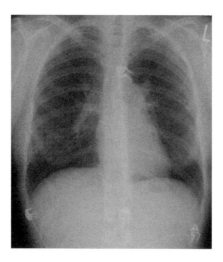

Fig. 2. Chest radiograph of a patient with severe pulmonary hypertension associated with MCTD. Note enlargement of bilateral pulmonary arteries.

controversial use of immunosuppressive medications in the treatment of PAH secondary to CTD.

Anticoagulation, oxygen, and diuretics

Two uncontrolled studies have demonstrated improved survival associated with the use of anticoagulation in patients with IPAH [30,31]. Anticoagulation has not been studied in patients with CTD-associated PAH but may be beneficial. Warfarin is considered the agent of choice for anticoagulation, and most experts recommend adjusting the dose to an international normalized ration of 1.5 to 2.5.

Hypoxia results in pulmonary arterial vasoconstriction, causing or worsening pulmonary hypertension. For this reason, supplemental oxygen is believed to be important in the treatment of PAH. No trials have been performed to assess the benefit of supplemental oxygen in the treatment of PAH secondary to CTD.

An important aspect of caring for patients who have severe pulmonary hypertension is careful regulation of their intravascular volume. Increased intravascular filling pressures can further distend an already dilated right ventricle, worsening its function and decreasing cardiac output. Diuretics should be used in patients with evidence of right heart failure, such as peripheral edema and ascites. Rapid diuresis is poorly tolerated by patients who have severe PAH and can lead to hypotension, renal insufficiency, and syncope. It is essential to instruct patients regarding the importance of sodium and fluid restrictions.

Vasodilators

Vasoconstriction of the pulmonary vascular bed is believed to play an important role in the pathobiology of severe pulmonary hypertension. The administration of pulmonary vasodilators is an important and evolving part of the treatment of patients with pulmonary hypertension. Many of these medications were initially used in the treatment of IPAH, and their role has expanded to include patients who have PAH associated with CTD.

Calcium-channel blockers

Oral calcium-channel blockers (CCBs) have been used in the treatment of PAH secondary to CTD, including patients who have MCTD. A landmark trial published by Rich and colleagues [30] in 1992 confirmed the benefit of CCBs in the treatment of a subset of patients who have IPAH. Patients who had a significant response (defined as a decrease in mean PA pressure of >20% and a decrease in pulmonary vascular resistance of >20%) to an acutely administered vasodilator (epoprostenol, adenosine, or inhaled NO) had improved 5-year survival when treated with oral CCBs compared with patients who did not respond acutely and with patients enrolled in the PPH NIH registry. It has been estimated that 5% to 20% of patients who have IPAH demonstrate this favorable response, and these patients may have up to a 94% survival rate at

5 years. There have been no randomized trials demonstrating the benefit of oral CCBs in patients who have PAH associated with CTD. There are a number of case reports and small case series reporting clinical and hemodynamic improvement in patients with scleroderma and MCTD treated with CCBs [32–35]. Although there are reports of improved outcomes in patients who have CTD treated with CCBs, it is generally believed that a small percentage of these patients responds favorably to this form of therapy. Other oral vasodilators, such as angiotensin inhibitors and alpha-adrenergic blockers, have been reported to be beneficial in small case series but have not been evaluated in a randomized fashion [33,36].

Prostanoids

Prostacyclin is a metabolite of arachidonic acid, produced primarily in the vascular endothelium [37–39]. It is a potent vasodilator that affects the pulmonary and systemic circulation. It has positive inotropic effects and inhibits platelet aggregation [40]. Chronic, continuous intravenous epoprostenol (also referred to as prostacyclin, prostaglandin I2, or Flolan) was the first drug approved by the FDA for the treatment of PAH [41–43]. It was initially approved for the treatment of IPAH patients with NYHA Class III and IV symptoms. The indication for this mediation was expanded to include patients who have significant PAH occurring in association with the scleroderma spectrum of diseases after a study by Badesch and colleagues [42] demonstrating its efficacy in this patient population. This study examined the efficacy of continuously infused epoprostenol in patients who have PAH associated with the "scleroderma spectrum of disease" as compared with conventional therapy. Fourteen percent of the patients in the treatment arm of this study were diagnosed with an "overlap syndrome" or MCTD. Epoprostenol was found to increase exercise capacity, hemodynamics, and clinical symptoms at 12 weeks. This study did not demonstrate a survival benefit but was underpowered to detect such a change.

Epoprostenol is difficult to receive and administer. It is unstable at pH values below 10.5. This, combined with its short half-life (3 minutes), prohibits oral administration; therefore, the drug must be given by continuous intravenous infusion. The requirement for permanent intravenous access places these patients at significant risk for catheter-related sepsis, which is poorly tolerated by patients with severe pulmonary hypertension.

Treprostinil

Treprostinil is a subcutaneously infused analog of prostacyclin. It has pharmacologic properties similar to those of epoprostenol with similar acute hemodynamic effects [44,45]. Treprostinil has the advantage of being chemically stable at room temperature and at a neutral pH. It also has a significantly longer half-life than epoprostenol (3–4 hours) and therefore can be administered subcutaneously via a microinfusion pump rather than intravenously. Treprostinil was demonstrated to be effective in the treatment of patients who had PAH in a double-blind, randomized, placebo-controlled trial [45]. A total of 470 patients were enrolled, including patients with IPAH or PAH associated with CTD or systemic-to-pulmonary arterial shunts. Treprostinil improved exercise capacity, Borg dyspnea score, and cardiopulmonary hemodynamics as assessed by cardiac catheterization. A survival benefit was not demonstrated. The most common side effect of this therapy was pain at the infusion site. Site pain led to discontinuation of therapy in 8% of patients [45]. Such discomfort can limit the ability to escalate the dose to effective levels. The efficacy and safety of treprostinil in treatment of PAH associated with CTD was readdressed in a study by Oudiz and colleagues [46]. In this study, 20% of the patients in the treatment arm and 18% of the patients in the placebo arm were diagnosed with MCTD. After 12 weeks, the patients who received treprostinil had significant improvements in 6-minute walk distance, hemodynamics, and dyspnea scores.

Endothelin antagonists

Endothlein-1 is a potent endogenous vasoconstrictor and is a smooth muscle mitogen. Endothelin-1 is overexpressed in the plasma and lung tissue of patients with IPAH and PAH related to scleroderma [47,48]. The actions of endothelin-1 are mediated by two receptors, ET_A and ET_B. ET_A, found predominantly on vascular smooth muscle cells, induces a vasoconstrictor effect. ET_B, which is found on endothelial cells and vascular smooth muscle, has a vasoconstrictor and vasodilator effect [49]. Medications have recently been developed that block these receptors.

Bosentan

Bosentan is an oral dual endothelin antagonist that blocks ET_A and ET_B receptors. Two randomized controlled trials have demonstrated the efficacy of bosentan in the treatment of PAH [47,48]. The Bosentan Randomized Trial of Endothelin Antagonist Therapy was a double-blind, placebo-controlled trial enrolling patients who had severe PAH (WHO functional class III or IV) who had IPAH or PAH associated with CTD (scleroderma or SLE) [48]. There was a significant improvement in 6-minute walk, the Borg dyspnea score, and time to clinical worsening in patients who received bosentan. There was no improvement in survival noted in either group. A follow-up study has shown that the clinical and hemodynamic benefits of bosentan therapy are maintained at 1 year [50]. Adverse affects of treatment with bosentan may include hepatotoxicity, anemia, fluid retention, teratogenicity, testicular atrophy, and male infertility. There is a significant risk of birth defects if bosentan is administered during pregnancy. In animal studies, bosentan induced malformations of the head, face, mouth, and vasculature. Infant mortality and miscarriages were increased in these studies. It is essential that pregnancy be excluded before therapy with bosentan is initiated. It is also important that hormonal therapy not be the sole means of contraception used during treatment with bosentan because a drug–drug interaction may occur, resulting in contraceptive failure. It is recommended that women of childbearing age have monthly pregnancy tests after initiating therapy with bosentan.

Because the ET_B receptor is involved in vasodilatation and in vasoconstriction, it has been postulated that blocking only the ET_A receptor may be clinically beneficial. With this in mind, two specific ET_A receptor blockers, Sitaxseten and Ambrisentan, have been developed and are being studied in randomized trials for the treatment of PAH.

Phosphodiesterase inhibitors

Recently, interest has surrounded a potential role for phosphodiesterase inhibitors in the treatment of PAH. Increased cellular levels of cyclic guanosine-monophosphate (cGMP) result in vasodilatation by relaxing vascular smooth muscle. Mediators such as NO raise levels of cGMP [51]. Conversely, phosphodiesterases degrade cGMP, facilitating vasoconstriction. The phosphodiesterase isoform active in degrading cGMP in the lung is cyclic nucleotide phosphodiesterase-5 (PDE-5) [52].

PDE-5 inhibitors cause pulmonary vasodilatation by inhibiting the degradation of cGMP. Sildenafil is a specific inhibitor of the phosphodiesterase isoform 5 and leads to smooth muscle relaxation via a NO-dependent increase of cGMP. A number of uncontrolled studies have suggested that the use of oral sildenafil may be beneficial in the treatment of PAH [53–55]. A small, open, controlled trial has demonstrated the potential benefit of adding sildenafil to the treatment of patients receiving continuous intravenous epoprostenol [56]. A larger, randomized, double-blind trial evaluating the use of sildenafil as monotherapy in the treatment of PAH has recently been completed. The results of this trial have not been published, but this drug will likely have a future role in the treatment of PAH associated with CTD.

Immunosuppressants

There are numerous reports of patients who have PAH associated with CTD improving clinically and hemodynamically after receiving immunosuppressive therapy [57–61]. However, there are no randomized controlled trials evaluating the efficacy of such therapy in these patients. Further confounding this issue, frequently the patients treated with immunosuppression also received vasodilator therapy. The immunosuppressive regimen and duration of therapy varied significantly between reported cases. For these reasons, it is difficult to make recommendations regarding the use of immunosuppressive therapy in the treatment of CTD-associated PAH in general or in MCTD in particular.

Other pulmonary manifestations of mixed connective tissue disease

Pleuropulmonary manifestations of MCTD are more common than previously recognized. The initial description of MCTD did not discuss pulmonary involvement of this disease. Subsequent publications have estimated that 20% to 80% of patients have respiratory involvement [1,62–64]. The potential respiratory manifestations of MCTD are listed in Box 1. Three of these respiratory diseases—interstitial disease, pleural effusions, and pulmonary hemorrhage—are discussed below.

Interstitial disease

The prevalence and incidence of interstitial lung disease in MCTD is poorly documented. Patients frequently present with complaints of dyspnea and non-productive cough, but abnormalities on pulmonary function tests and chest radiographs are common in asymptomatic patients as well. Up to one third of patients who have MCTD have abnormal chest radiographs, frequently demonstrating interstitial changes in the lung bases [64]. Changes characteristic of MCTD seen on high-resolution CT include ground-glass attenuation and non-septal linear opacities with a peripheral and lower lobe predominance [65]. There is little published literature regarding the histology of interstitial lung disease associated with MCTD. It is speculated that the major lung injury patterns include nonspecific interstitial pneumonitis and usual interstitial pneumonitis. Treatment involves corticosteroid or immunosuppressive therapy, but there is no definitive proof that such therapy affects outcome.

Pleural disease

Pleural manifestations of CTD are common, and MCTD is no exception. The overall incidence of pleural effusion in MCTD has been estimated to be as high as 50%. Occasionally, pleural disease can be the presenting symptom of MCTD [66]. Prakash and colleagues [62,63] reported on the intrathoracic manifestations of 81 patients who had MCTD. In this series, 6% of the patients had pleural effusions, and 2% had pleural thickening. However, in a series of 34 patients presented by Sullivan and colleagues [64], 40% had pleuritic chest pain. The effusions are frequently exudative in nature and are often self-limited.

Alveolar hemorrhage

SLE has a well-recognized association with pulmonary alveolar hemorrhage [67]. There are case reports of patients who have MCTD presenting with alveolar hemorrhage. Germain et al [68] described a patient who had MCTD who developed pulmonary hemorrhage and acute renal failure. Schwarz and colleagues [69] reported on a case of diffuse alveolar hemorrhage due to capillaritis in a patient who had MCTD. The etiology of alveolar hemorrhage in MCTD is unclear, although it is presumably similar in etiology to that seen in SLE and may involve immune complex deposition. There are no trials to direct therapy of this potentially life-threatening manifestation of MCTD, but many experts support the use of anti-inflammatory or immune-suppressive agents. The role of plasmapheresis is unclear [67].

References

[1] Sharp GC, Irvin WS, May CM, et al. Association of antibodies to ribonucleoprotein and Sm antigens with mixed connective-tissue disease, systematic lupus erythematosus and other rheumatic diseases. N Engl J Med 1976;295:1149–54.
[2] Rubin LJ. Primary pulmonary hypertension. N Engl J Med 1997;336:111–7.
[3] Dorfmuller P, Perros F, Balabanian K, et al. Inflammation in pulmonary arterial hypertension. Eur Respir J 2003;22:358–63.
[4] Chu JW, Kao PN, Faul JL, et al. High prevalence of autoimmune thyroid disease in pulmonary arterial hypertension. Chest 2002;122:1668–73.
[5] Morse JH, Barst RJ, Fotino M, et al. Primary pulmonary hypertension, tissue plasminogen activator antibodies, and HLA-DQ7. Am J Respir Crit Care Med 1997;155:274–8.
[6] Asherson RA, Harris EN, Bernstein RM, et al. Immunological studies in 'primary' idiopathic pulmonary hypertension. Eur J Rheumatol Inflamm 1984;7:75–9.
[7] Barst RJ, Loyd JE. Genetics and immunogenetic aspects of primary pulmonary hypertension. Chest 1998;114(Suppl):231S–6S.
[8] Young RH, Mark GJ. Pulmonary vascular changes in scleroderma. Am J Med 1978;64: 998–1004.
[9] Cool CD, Kennedy D, Voelkel NF, et al. Pathogenesis and evolution of plexiform lesions in pulmonary hypertension associated with scleroderma and human immunodeficiency virus infection. Hum Pathol 1997;28:434–42.
[10] Quismorio Jr FP, Sharma O, Koss M, et al. Immunopathologic and clinical studies in pulmonary hypertension associated with systemic lupus erythematosus. Semin Arthritis Rheum 1984;13: 349–59.
[11] Yeo PP, Sinniah R. Lupus cor pulmonale with electron microscope and immunofluorescent antibody studies. Ann Rheum Dis 1975;34:457–60.
[12] Asherson RA, Hackett D, Gharavi AE, et al. Pulmonary hypertension in systemic lupus erythematosus: a report of three cases. J Rheumatol 1986;13:416–20.
[13] Asherson RA, Oakley CM. Pulmonary hypertension and systemic lupus erythematosus. J Rheumatol 1986;13:1–5.
[14] Stupi AM, Steen VD, Owens GR, et al. Pulmonary hypertension in the CREST syndrome variant of systemic sclerosis. Arthritis Rheum 1986;29:515–24.
[15] Li EK, Tam LS. Pulmonary hypertension in systemic lupus erythematosus: clinical association and survival in 18 patients. J Rheumatol 1999;26:1923–9.
[16] Fahey PJ, Utell MJ, Condemi JJ, et al. Raynaud's phenomenon of the lung. Am J Med 1984;76:263–9.
[17] Rozkovec A, Bernstein R, Asherson RA, et al. Vascular reactivity and pulmonary hypertension in systemic sclerosis. Arthritis Rheum 1983;26:1037–40.
[18] Seoane L, Shellito J, Welsh D, et al. Pulmonary hypertension associated with HIV infection. South Med J 2001;94:635–9.
[19] Pellicelli AM, Barbaro G, Palmieri F, et al. Primary pulmonary hypertension in HIV patients: a systematic review. Angiology 2001;52:31–41.
[20] Bull TM, Cool CD, Serls AE, et al. Primary pulmonary hypertension, Castleman's disease and human herpesvirus-8. Eur Respir J 2003;22:403–7.

[21] Cool CD, Rai PR, Yeager ME, et al. Expression of human herpesvirus 8 in primary pulmonary hypertension. N Engl J Med 2003;349:1113–22.

[22] Deng Z, Morse JH, Slager SL, et al. Familial primary pulmonary hypertension (gene PPH1) is caused by mutations in the bone morphogenetic protein receptor-II gene. Am J Hum Genet 2000;67:737–44.

[23] Machado RD, Pauciulo MW, Thomson JR, et al. BMPR2 Haploinsufficiency as the inherited molecular mechanism for primary pulmonary hypertension. Am J Hum Genet 2001;68:92–102.

[24] Thomson JR, Machado RD, Pauciulo MW, et al. Sporadic primary pulmonary hypertension is associated with germline mutations of the gene encoding BMPR-II, a receptor member of the TGF-beta family. J Med Genet 2000;37:741–5.

[25] Tew MB, Arnett FC, Reveille JD, et al. Mutations of bone morphogenetic protein receptor type II are not found in patients with pulmonary hypertension and underlying connective tissue diseases. Arthritis Rheum 2002;46:2829–30.

[26] Morse J, Barst R, Horn E, et al. Pulmonary hypertension in scleroderma spectrum of disease: lack of bone morphogenetic protein receptor 2 mutations. J Rheumatol 2002;29:2379–81.

[27] Esther JH, Sharp GC, Agia G, et al. Pulmonary hypertension in patients with connective tissue disease and antibody to nuclear ribonucleoprotein. Arthritis Rheum 1981;24:S105.

[28] Wiener-Kronish JP, Solinger AM, Warnock ML, et al. Severe pulmonary involvement in mixed connective tissue disease. Am Rev Respir Dis 1981;124:499–503.

[29] Hosoda Y, Suzuki Y, Takano M, et al. Mixed connective tissue disease with pulmonary hypertension: a clinical and pathological study. J Rheumatol 1987;14:826–30.

[30] Rich S, Kaufmann E, Levy PS. The effect of high doses of calcium-channel blockers on survival in primary pulmonary hypertension. N Engl J Med 1992;327:76–81.

[31] Fuster V, Steele PM, Edwards WD, et al. Primary pulmonary hypertension: natural history and the importance of thrombosis. Circulation 1984;70:580–7.

[32] Alpert MA, Pressly TA, Mukerji V, et al. Acute and long-term effects of nifedipine on pulmonary and systemic hemodynamics in patients with pulmonary hypertension associated with diffuse systemic sclerosis, the CREST syndrome and mixed connective tissue disease. Am J Cardiol 1991;68:1687–91.

[33] Glikson M, Pollack A, Dresner-Feigin R, et al. Nifedipine and prazosin in the management of pulmonary hypertension in CREST syndrome. Chest 1990;98:759–61.

[34] O'Brien JT, Hill JA, Pepine CJ. Sustained benefit of verapamil in pulmonary hypertension with progressive systemic sclerosis. Am Heart J 1985;109:380–2.

[35] Sfikakis PP, Kyriakidis MK, Vergos CG, et al. Cardiopulmonary hemodynamics in systemic sclerosis and response to nifedipine and captopril. Am J Med 1991;90:541–6.

[36] Alpert MA, Pressly TA, Mukerji V, et al. Short- and long-term hemodynamic effects of captopril in patients with pulmonary hypertension and selected connective tissue disease. Chest 1992;102:1407–12.

[37] Dusting GJ, Moncada S, Vane JR. Prostacyclin: its biosynthesis, actions, and clinical potential. Adv Prostaglandin Thromboxane Leukot Res 1982;10:59–106.

[38] Geraci M, Gao B, Shepherd D, et al. Pulmonary prostacyclin synthase overexpression by adenovirus transfection and in transgenic mice. Chest 1998;114(Suppl):99S.

[39] Brock TG, McNish RW, Peters-Golden M. Arachidonic acid is preferentially metabolized by cyclooxygenase-2 to prostacyclin and prostaglandin E2. J Biol Chem 1999;274:11660–6.

[40] Weir EK, Rubin LJ, Ayres SM, et al. The acute administration of vasodilators in primary pulmonary hypertension: experience from the National Institutes of Health Registry on Primary Pulmonary Hypertension. Am Rev Respir Dis 1989;140:1623–30.

[41] Rubin LJ, Mendoza J, Hood M, et al. Treatment of primary pulmonary hypertension with continuous intravenous prostacyclin (epoprostenol): results of a randomized trial. Ann Intern Med 1990;112:485–91.

[42] Badesch DB, Tapson VF, McGoon MD, et al. Continuous intravenous epoprostenol for pulmonary hypertension due to the scleroderma spectrum of disease: a randomized, controlled trial. Ann Intern Med 2000;132:425–34.

[43] Barst RJ, Rubin LJ, Long WA, et al. A comparison of continuous intravenous epoprostenol (prostacyclin) with conventional therapy for primary pulmonary hypertension. The Primary Pulmonary Hypertension Study Group. N Engl J Med 1996;334:296–302.

[44] McNulty MJ, Sailstad JM, Steffen RP. The pharmacokinetics and pharmacodynamics of the prostacyclin analog 15AU81 in the anesthetized beagle dog. Prostaglandins Leukot Essent Fatty Acids 1993;48:159–66.

[45] Simonneau G, Barst RJ, Galie N, et al. Continuous subcutaneous infusion of treprostinil, a prostacyclin analogue, in patients with pulmonary arterial hypertension: a double- blind, randomized, placebo-controlled trial. Am J Respir Crit Care Med 2002;165:800–4.

[46] Oudiz RJ, Schilz RJ, Barst RJ, et al. Treprostinil, a prostacyclin analogue, in pulmonary arterial hypertension associated with connective tissue disease. Chest 2004;126:420–7.

[47] Channick RN, Simonneau G, Sitbon O, et al. Effects of the dual endothelin-receptor antagonist bosentan in patients with pulmonary hypertension: a randomised placebo-controlled study. Lancet 2001;358:1119–23.

[48] Rubin LJ, Badesch DB, Barst RJ, et al. Bosentan therapy for pulmonary arterial hypertension. N Engl J Med 2002;346:896–903.

[49] Kim NH, Rubin LJ. Endothelin in health and disease: endothelin receptor antagonists in the management of pulmonary artery hypertension. J Cardiovasc Pharmacol Ther 2002;7:9–19.

[50] Sitbon O, Badesch DB, Channick RN, et al. Effects of the dual endothelin receptor antagonist bosentan in patients with pulmonary arterial hypertension: a 1-year follow-up study. Chest 2003;124:247–54.

[51] Murad F. Cyclic GMP: synthesis, metabolism, and function. Introduction and some historical comments. Adv Pharmacol 1994;26:1–5.

[52] Gibson A. Phosphodiesterase 5 inhibitors and nitrergic transmission-from zaprinast to sildenafil. Eur J Pharmacol 2001;411:1–10.

[53] Michelakis E, Tymchak W, Lien D, et al. Oral sildenafil is an effective and specific pulmonary vasodilator in patients with pulmonary arterial hypertension: comparison with inhaled nitric oxide. Circulation 2002;105:2398–403.

[54] Abrams D, Schulze-Neick I, Magee AG. Sildenafil as a selective pulmonary vasodilator in childhood primary pulmonary hypertension. Heart 2000;84:E4.

[55] Prasad S, Wilkinson J, Gatzoulis MA. Sildenafil in primary pulmonary hypertension. N Engl J Med 2000;343:1342.

[56] Stiebellehner L, Petkov V, Vonbank K, et al. Long-term treatment with oral sildenafil in addition to continuous IV epoprostenol in patients with pulmonary arterial hypertension. Chest 2003; 123:1293–5.

[57] Karmochkine M, Wechsler B, Godeau P, et al. Improvement of severe pulmonary hypertension in a patient with SLE. Ann Rheum Dis 1996;55:561–2.

[58] Morelli S, Giordano M, De Marzio P, et al. Pulmonary arterial hypertension responsive to immunosuppressive therapy in systemic lupus erythematosus. Lupus 1993;2:367–9.

[59] Groen H, Bootsma H, Postma DS, et al. Primary pulmonary hypertension in a patient with systemic lupus erythematosus: partial improvement with cyclophosphamide. J Rheumatol 1993; 20:1055–7.

[60] Goupille P, Fauchier L, Babuty D, et al. Precapillary pulmonary hypertension dramatically improved with high doses of corticosteroids during systemic lupus erythematosus. J Rheumatol 1994;21:1976–7.

[61] Dahl M, Chalmers A, Wade J, et al. Ten year survival of a patient with advanced pulmonary hypertension and mixed connective tissue disease treated with immunosuppressive therapy. J Rheumatol 1992;19:1807–9.

[62] Prakash UB. Respiratory complications in mixed connective tissue disease. Clin Chest Med 1998;19:733–46.

[63] Prakash UB, Luthra HS, Divertie MB. Intrathoracic manifestations in mixed connective tissue disease. Mayo Clin Proc 1985;60:813–21.

[64] Sullivan WD, Hurst DJ, Harmon CE, et al. A prospective evaluation emphasizing pulmonary

involvement in patients with mixed connective tissue disease. Medicine (Baltimore) 1984;63: 92–107.

[65] Kozuka T, Johkoh T, Honda O, et al. Pulmonary involvement in mixed connective tissue disease: high-resolution CT findings in 41 patients. J Thorac Imaging 2001;16:94–8.

[66] Hoogsteden HC, van Dongen JJ, van der Kwast TH, et al. Bilateral exudative pleuritis, an unusual pulmonary onset of mixed connective tissue disease. Respiration (Herrlisheim) 1985;48: 164–7.

[67] Zamora MR, Warner ML, Tuder R, et al. Diffuse alveolar hemorrhage and systemic lupus erythematosus: clinical presentation, histology, survival, and outcome. Medicine (Baltimore) 1997;76:192–202.

[68] Germain MJ, Davidman M. Pulmonary hemorrhage and acute renal failure in a patient with mixed connective tissue disease. Am J Kidney Dis 1984;3:420–4.

[69] Schwarz MI, Zamora MR, Hodges TN, et al. Isolated pulmonary capillaritis and diffuse alveolar hemorrhage in rheumatoid arthritis and mixed connective tissue disease. Chest 1998;113: 1609–15.

ELSEVIER
SAUNDERS

RHEUMATIC
DISEASE CLINICS
OF NORTH AMERICA

Rheum Dis Clin N Am 31 (2005) 465–481

Raynaud's Phenomenon in Mixed Connective Tissue Disease

Thomas Grader-Beck, MD, PhD, Fredrick M. Wigley, MD*

Division of Rheumatology, Johns Hopkins School of Medicine, 5200 Eastern Avenue, Suite 4100, Baltimore, MD 21224, USA

When Sharp and colleagues [1] first identified the mixed connective tissue disease (MCTD) phenotype, it was based solely on serologic evidence that was characterized by high-titer autoantibodies to U1-RNP (ribonucleoprotein). Although the clinical phenotype included overlapping symptoms of systemic lupus erythematosus (SLE), scleroderma, and polymyositis to various degrees, it was striking that Raynaud's phenomenon was a dominant symptom in all of these patients. Eighty-four percent of patients in this initial group was suffering from Raynaud's phenomenon. It often is the first symptom; long-term follow-up of patients who have MCTD suggests that symptoms of Raynaud's phenomenon remain constant over time [2]. As a consequence, Raynaud's phenomenon is included as a major criterion in Sharp and colleagues' proposal [1] for a diagnosis of MCTD. A high frequency of Raynaud's phenomenon in MCTD was confirmed subsequently by other investigators [3–6]. Raynaud's phenomenon has maintained its importance as part of two current alternative sets of diagnostic criteria for MCTD that were proposed by Alarçon-Segovia and Kasukawa [7]. Although the existence of MCTD as a distinct disease entity has remained a matter of debate, Raynaud's phenomenon represents a dominant symptom in patients who have the clinical phenotype that meets current diagnostic criteria.

Raynaud's phenomenon is characterized by episodes of ischemia, which most commonly involves the digits of the hands and feet and leads to typical dual or tricolor skin changes. Episodes are triggered by exposure to cold or emotional stress. It is common for patients to experience numbness, pain, and paresthesias during the ischemia which is caused by digital vasospasm. Raynaud's phenome-

---

* Corresponding author.
E-mail address: fwig@jhmi.edu (F.M. Wigley).

0889-857X/05/$ – see front matter © 2005 Elsevier Inc. All rights reserved.
doi:10.1016/j.rdc.2005.04.006
rheumatic.theclinics.com

non may just be the manifestation of an exaggerated response of the cutaneous thermoregulatory vessels and digital arteries to cold, stress, or trauma, or it can be associated with a disease state, such as MCTD.

Primary Raynaud's phenomenon is characterized by the absence of an underlying systemic disorder and represents a common symptom in the general population; it is observed in approximately 3% to 5% of individuals in the United States [8–10]. A frequent cause of secondary Raynaud's phenomenon is an underlying systemic rheumatic disease. It is estimated that approximately 21% to 44% of patients who have SLE [11,12], 13% of patients who have primary Sjögren's syndrome [13], up to 17% of patients who have rheumatoid arthritis [14], and approximately 10% of patients who have polymyositis suffer from Raynaud's phenomenon. Furthermore, patients who have undifferentiated connective tissue disease (UCTD) demonstrate a high prevalence (~50%) of Raynaud's phenomenon [15,16]. The highest prevalence of Raynaud's phenomenon is observed among patients who have systemic sclerosis (scleroderma) and MCTD and approaches 90% or greater in most studies [17–20].

One of the challenges that faces the physician who encounters a patient who has Raynaud's phenomenon is to determine whether there is a secondary cause for the problem. Raynaud's phenomenon is a common initial symptom in patients who go on to develop MCTD, yet on presentation, they may not have other features of the disease or meet classification criteria. For example, one case series showed that in 15 patients who had MCTD and were suffering from Raynaud's phenomenon, it was the initial symptom in 14 patients [5].

The first part of this article discusses several clinical and serologic aspects of the patient who presents with Raynaud's phenomenon that should raise the suspicion that he/she may evolve into an MCTD phenotype. This is followed by a discussion about the extent to which Raynaud's phenomenon in MCTD is the clinical manifestation of a unique pathophysiologic process. The final part of the article focuses on therapeutic considerations.

It is important to acknowledge the obstacles that the authors encountered when reviewing the literature on Raynaud's phenomenon in MCTD. These include: (1) the presence of different sets of diagnostic criteria for MCTD that were used in studies (eg, Sharp [22], Alarcón-Segovia and Villareal [7], Kasukawa and colleagues [21], and Kahn and colleagues [23]); (2) the heterogeneity of assays that are used to detect the autoantibody U1-RNP and its components—the autoantibody that is one of the accepted requirements for the diagnosis of MCTD; (3) the evolution of a significant percentage of cases of MCTD into another rheumatic disease (eg, scleroderma, SLE, polymyositis); and finally, (4) the ongoing debate as to whether MCTD represents a distinct disease entity, and consequently, a failure to classify these patients accordingly.

Nevertheless, when faced with a patient who has Raynaud's phenomenon, the authors believe that there are characteristic findings, including capillary nailfold changes defined by microscopy, autoantibody specificity, and clinical features, that will identify patients who are at risk of developing the MCTD phenotype.

Capillary nailfold studies

Nailfold capillary microscopy has been advocated as a valuable tool by many investigators to differentiate primary from secondary Raynaud's phenomenon. Several studies have demonstrated that patients who have primary Raynaud's phenomenon do not exhibit capillary nailfold changes [24–26]. Conversely, patients who have MCTD, scleroderma, and dermatomyositis demonstrate characteristic nailfold capillary abnormalities. Maricq [27] described two different types of scleroderma pattern: slow and active. Irregularly enlarged or giant loops with no or minimal capillary loss is characteristic of the slow pattern, whereas the active pattern demonstrates definite capillary loss and general disorganization and neoformation of capillaries [27]. Patients who have MCTD demonstrate characteristic abnormalities on nailfold capillary microscopy that typically resemble the slow scleroderma pattern. In particular, giant or megacapillaries and nailfold hemorrhages are characteristic changes. In one study, more than 63% of patients who had MCTD demonstrated a scleroderma-like pattern, with bushy capillaries being a dominant feature [4]. Megacapillaries are another dominant feature that was observed in 56% of patients who had MCTD [28]. Patients who have MCTD also may demonstrate mostly avascular areas that surround enlarged and deformed capillary loops [29].

Therefore, patients who present with Raynaud's phenomenon alone should undergo careful nailfold capillary examination. If a slow scleroderma pattern is present, then MCTD should be included in the differential diagnosis.

Capillary nailfold changes in patients who have MCTD are characteristic, particularly when compared with patients who have SLE. Despite a similar high frequency of Raynaud's phenomenon in SLE versus MCTD in one study, only 2% of patients who had SLE exhibited a scleroderma-like pattern compared with 54% of patients who had MCTD [29]. A similar observation was made in another study [4]. When patients who have SLE have MCTD-like capillary abnormalities, they are more likely to have U1-RNP autoantibodies [30]. One group of investigators demonstrated that abnormal capillary loops (wider caliber and broader loops) were observed in only 3 of 19 patients who had SLE [31]. Strikingly, all 3 patients had anti–U1-RNP autoantibodies, although 1 did not suffer from Raynaud's phenomenon.

Raynaud's phenomenon and anti–U1-ribonucleoprotein

Because Raynaud's phenomenon is common among patients who have MCTD, and high titer autoantibodies against U1-RNP are a requirement for the diagnosis of MCTD, it is conceivable that U1-RNP autoantibodies may represent a marker for the vascular process that causes Raynaud's phenomenon or that these antibodies play a causal role in the associated structural vasculopathy. Although it initially was believed that only patients with anti-U1-RNP have true MCTD, subsequent studies revealed that up to 29% of patients who had UCTD

[15], up to 21% of patients who had scleroderma [32], and 25% to 30% of patients who had SLE [33,34] also develop antibodies to U1-RNP. Several studies demonstrate an intimate relationship between Raynaud's phenomenon and the presence of anti-U1-RNP in these patient populations. There also is evidence that these populations may share a similar risk of developing specific visceral complications (Fig. 1).

A relationship between anti-U1-RNP positivity and Raynaud's phenomenon in UCTD was reported in several studies [16,35,36]. Patients who had UCTD and Raynaud's phenomenon had a threefold greater prevalence of U1-RNP positivity and approximately a tenfold greater prevalence of esophageal dysmotility compared with patients who did not have Raynaud's phenomenon [15]. Anti–U1-RNP positivity correlated with a slow scleroderma pattern by nailfold capillary microscopy.

In a large study of 276 consecutive patients who had scleroderma, antibodies to U1-RNP were demonstrated in more than 21% of patients [32]; 90% of those patients had Raynaud's phenomenon. Pulmonary complications were frequent; 86% demonstrated a decrease in DLCO, and overt pulmonary hypertension was evident in 48%. In a different study, 18 of 223 (8%) patients who had scleroderma were positive for anti–U1-RNP and uniformly demonstrated Raynaud's phenomenon [37]. These patients had a twofold greater incidence of pulmonary fibrosis and a threefold greater incidence of decreased vital capacity

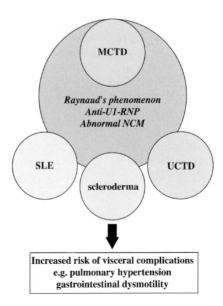

Fig. 1. A common phenotype across the spectrum of systemic rheumatic diseases. Patients who present with Raynaud's phenomenon in the presence of U1-RNP (ribonucleoprotein) autoantibodies and capillary nailfold abnormalities have a higher risk for developing similar visceral complications, including pulmonary hypertension and gastrointestinal dysmotility, regardless of the underlying disease. NCM, nailfold capillary microscopy.

compared with their U1-RNP negative counterparts. In another study, Raynaud's phenomenon was found in almost all anti-U1-RNP positive patients who had scleroderma and was associated with a greater incidence of pulmonary hypertension [38].

A recent European multicenter prospective study of 289 patients who had SLE found that anti-U1-RNP positive patients have the highest odds ratio for Raynaud's phenomenon compared with other autoantibodies that are found in SLE [39]. Other investigators observed that anti–U1-RNP positive patients who had SLE had a much greater likelihood of Raynaud's phenomenon, interstitial changes on chest radiogram, and decreased capillary loops [40]. An increased prevalence of Raynaud's phenomenon that was associated with a decrease in DLCO in anti–U1-RNP positive patients who had SLE was confirmed in another study [41].

These studies suggest that patients who have a clinical diagnosis of SLE and have Raynaud's phenomenon with the nailfold capillary changes that are seen in scleroderma represent a unique SLE subset that is at risk for pulmonary disease, particularly in the setting of anti–U1-RNP positivity. It is possible that the fine specificity of U1-RNP reactivity may help to identify this subset of patients who have SLE further. Patients who have MCTD typically recognize the U1-70K protein as well as protein A and C, all of which represent unique structures of the U1-RNP complex [42]. Anti–U1-RNP positive patients who have scleroderma or MCTD demonstrate a several fold greater positivity for U1-70K protein compared with U1-RNP positive patients who have SLE [43,44]; persistent U1-70K specificity has been associated with death from pulmonary hypertension in patients who have MCTD [2]. Therefore, the U1-70K positive patient population that has SLE is at a particularly high risk for developing the MCTD phenotype. In addition, although most U1-RNP positive patients who have SLE demonstrate concomitant autoantibodies to Sm (dual-specificity), it may be that the monospecific anti–U1-RNP positive population that has SLE more closely resembles the MCTD phenotype, including Raynaud's and pulmonary complications; however, studies are needed to address these questions.

These observations support the conclusion that anti-U1-RNP positivity strongly correlates with the presence of Raynaud's phenomenon and pulmonary disease, especially pulmonary hypertension, across a wide spectrum of connective tissue diseases including MCTD, SLE, scleroderma, and possibly, UCTD (see Fig. 1).

Pathogenesis of Raynaud's phenomenon in mixed connective tissue disease

Despite recent advances, the pathogenesis of Raynaud's phenomenon remains incompletely understood. Although primary Raynaud's phenomenon is widely considered to be restricted to reversible vasospasm, there is evidence that in secondary Raynaud's phenomenon a concomitant structural vasculopathy contributes to the disease process. In the authors' experience, Raynaud's phenomenon tends to be less severe in patients who have MCTD than in patients who have scleroderma, including a lower frequency of digital ulcers or loss of digits. There are no reliable predictors that identify patients who have MCTD who are at risk for developing severe complications from Raynaud's phenomenon. In patients who have scleroderma, anticentromere positivity confers a higher risk of ischemic digital loss [45], and recognition of a specific centromere fragment that is created by granzyme B cleavage is associated with ischemic digital loss [46]. Conversely, in most patients who have SLE, Raynaud's phenomenon seems to involve different processes, unless they have anti-U1 RNP antibodies and scleroderma-like nailfold capillary changes. In the latter group, Raynaud's phenomenon is more severe and those patients are more likely to have digital ischemic events. The characteristic capillary nailfold changes that are observed in MCTD, scleroderma, and some cases of SLE suggest a similar pathophysiologic process among these patient groups.

Much of our current understanding of secondary Raynaud's phenomenon is derived from studies in scleroderma. The vasculopathy in scleroderma consists of diffuse intimal fibrosis in small and medium arteries, activation of smooth muscle cells, and endothelial cell perturbations. Smooth muscle cells of small cutaneous vessels from patients who have scleroderma demonstrate an increase in α2-adrenergic responsiveness even before there is evidence of endothelial dysfunction [47]. One hypothesis is that intimal hyperplasia is a consequence of activation and differentiation of vascular smooth muscle cells into myofibroblasts that secrete excess amounts of extracellular matrix. Another theory is that there is an influx of primitive stem cells into the intimal layer where they secrete collagen and other extracellular matrix components in an attempt to repair vascular damage. The process of intimal fibrosis progressively narrows the lumen of the affected vessels, prevents normal blood flow, and causes chronic tissue hypoxia. The evidence also demonstrates that the vascular disease of scleroderma, and likely MCTD, is associated with endothelial activation and subsequent platelet activation. Factors that are released from the disturbed endothelial cell layer and activated platelets compromise local blood flow, and lead to intimal fibrosis and local thrombosis. High levels of von Willebrand factor antigen and ristomycin-cofactor activity have been found in patients who have MCTD; this indicates that platelet activation may play a role in the vasculopathy [48].

A review of studies in MCTD suggests similarities to the vasculopathy in scleroderma spectrum disorders. Sharp and colleagues [1], in their initial description, noted that 6 out of 10 patients who had skin biopsies had changes that were consistent with scleroderma. In another study, forearm skin samples from patients who had MCTD demonstrated inflammatory cell infiltration around the small vessels in the papillary layer, intimal thickening of small arteries, and organized thrombus of the veins [49]. Patients who have MCTD exhibit a significant increase in basal membrane layering with greater layering of pericytes and laminae in muscle biopsies compared with patients who have SLE alone [50]. Similar electron microscopy findings were noted in capillary nailfold biopsies [51]. Patients who had MCTD in this study demonstrated a similar percentage of mast cells and activated or increased fibroblasts as patients who had scleroderma, whereas none of the patients who had SLE showed this abnormality. Skin biopsies of several patients who had MCTD and skin involvement that was typical of subacute cutaneous lupus erythematous showed clear evidence of a microangiopathy [52]; typically, this is not observed in patients who have SLE. A striking reduction in the superficial vascular plexus density, along with vascular ectasia was noted. Thrombogenic vasculopathy was found in one case and complement deposition in two cases. Autopsy examination of cases of MCTD revealed widespread proliferative vascular lesions in the intima and media of muscular-type arteries and arterioles [53–56]. Patients who have MCTD also demonstrate an increased prevalence of macrovascular disease with obstruction of ulnar, palmar arch, and digital arteries [57]. This pattern also is observed characteristically in patients who have limited scleroderma [58].

Recent evidence suggests that the autoantibodies that are found in patients who have MCTD may contribute to the development of the vasculopathy. Autoantibodies may cause damage to the vessel wall in several ways, including (1) binding of endothelial cell targets and subsequent activation or apoptosis, (2) binding to extracellular matrix structures after the endothelium is injured, and (3) deposition of immune complexes and complement activation within the vessel wall. It has been postulated that activation or apoptosis of endothelial cells could lead to the release of vasoconstrictors (eg, endothelin) and the underproduction of vasodilators, including prostacyclin and nitric oxide. In line with this hypothesis, antiendothelial cell antibodies (AECAs) have been found in high frequency in patients who have scleroderma and can induce endothelial cell apoptosis [59]. Similarly, up to 45% of patients who have MCTD demonstrate serum AECAs [60]. Up-regulation of serum AECAs in the setting of active MCTD was described recently [61]. Purified immunoglobulin from these patients increased E-selectin expression on cultured human umbilical vein endothelial cells.

U1-RNP antibodies may contribute directly to the vasculopathy that is observed in patients who have MCTD. A series of studies from one group demonstrated that antibodies to U1-RNP stimulate cytokine secretion from mononuclear cells and induce an increase in the expression of adhesion cell molecules, intercellular adhesion molecule–1 and endothelial leukocyte adhesion molecule–1, and major histocompatibility complex class II on human pulmonary artery endothelial cells (HPAECs). Direct binding of anti-RNP IgG and F_{ab} fragments were demonstrated on cultured HPAECs [62–65]. Whether a similar process occurs in vivo and in digital arteries of patients who have MCTD with Raynaud's phenomenon is conceivable but remains speculative.

Other autoantibodies also may be associated with MCTD, although their pathogenic role is uncertain. Fibrillin-1 is expressed in arterial and venous walls, where it fulfills load-bearing and anchoring functions. It can be produced by cultured endothelial cells [66] and is abundant in vascular subendothelium where it may be targeted by anti–fibrillin-1–specific autoantibodies. Anti–fibrillin-1 IgG autoantibodies were found in 34% of patients who had MCTD and white patients who had scleroderma, but only in 1% of patients who had SLE [67]. There was no cross-reaction between antitopoisomerase I, anticentromere, and anti-RNA polymerase antibodies. A high percentage (47%) of anti–fibrillin-1 positive patients who had MCTD was confirmed in a subsequent study [68]. No clear association between disease activity and autoantibody titer was observed.

The approach to therapy of Raynaud's phenomenon in mixed connective tissue disease

The vasculopathy in MCTD resembles that of scleroderma to a high degree, and therefore, the clinical consequences are similar. These patients exhibit several components of vascular abnormalities, including (1) recurrent episodes of vasospasm (Raynaud's phenomenon); (2) a structural disease component that includes intimal fibrosis and narrowing of the vessel lumen; and (3) the potential for formation of intravascular thrombi. Therefore, therapy should be tailored to prevent and reverse each of these individual components. The goal is to decrease the frequency of attacks, prevent digital ulceration, and to limit progressive vascular damage because complete abrogation of Raynaud's phenomenon is observed rarely with current available therapy. Although nondrug therapy is the most effective mode of treatment, one can argue that all patients also should be treated with medications, even in the absence of digital ulcers. This is especially true because it is believed that recurrent ischemia-reperfusion injury contributes to the structural vasculopathy over time. Certainly, no one would argue that patients who have digital ulcers should be treated aggressively.

Nondrug therapy

All patients should be instructed to keep their whole body warm and to avoid aggravating factors, such as stress, digital trauma, and medications that lead to vasoconstriction. The frequency and severity of Raynaud's attacks are temperature-dependent as shown by the difference in digital complications in the winter compared with the summer. There is no more effective therapy for Raynaud's phenomenon than avoiding cold or rapidly shifting temperatures.

Drug therapy

Vasodilators

The standard drug therapy for patients who have MCTD and Raynaud's phenomenon is a calcium channel blocker (Fig. 2). The dihydropyridine class of agents are potent vasodilators and are efficacious in the treatment of Raynaud's phenomenon. On average, a moderate reduction in the frequency of attacks and a

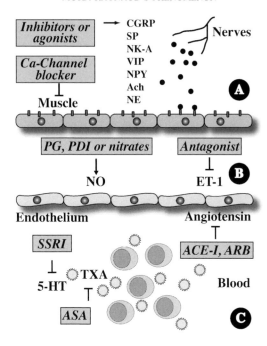

Fig. 2. Regulators of blood vessel tone and therapeutic approaches for Raynaud's phenomenon. (*A*) The nerve–muscle interface represents a complex interface of neuropeptide-mediated regulation of blood vessel tone. Calcium (Ca) channel blockers inhibit smooth muscle contraction. Agonists and inhibitors of neuromediators are being investigated for the therapy of Raynauds's phenomenon. ACE-inhibitors (ACE-I) and angiotensin-II receptor blockers (ARB) inhibit angiotensin-mediated vasoconstriction and may have a protective endothelial effect. (*B*) Endothelin-1 (ET-1) is a potent vasoconstrictor and mitogen for endothelial and smooth muscle cells. Its action is inhibited by endothelin receptor antagonists (eg, bosentan). Prostaglandin (PG) analogs, such as iloprost and epoprostenol, are potent vasodilators that facilitate the release of vasodilatory nitric oxide (NO), and additionally inhibit platelet aggregation and stimulate fibrinolysis. NO release is stimulated by phosphodiesterase inhibitors (PDI) and nitrates. (*C*) Platelet activation leads to intraluminal release of the potent vasoconstrictors thromboxane A (TXA) and serotonin. Synthesis of TXA by platelets is inhibited by aspirin (ASA), whereas serotonin-reuptake inhibitors (SSRI) reduce circulating levels of serotonin and its uptake into platelets. 5-HT, 5-Hydroxytryptophan; Ach, actetylcholine; CGRP, calcitonin-gene related peptide; NE, norepinephrine; NK-A, neurokinin A; NPY, neuropeptide Y; SP, substance P; VIP, vasointestinal peptide.

35% improvement of severity can be expected, according to a recent meta-analysis of patients who had scleroderma [69]. Although nifedipine has been studied most extensively, the newer dihydropyridines, including felodipine, amlodipine, and isradipine, seem to be equally effective [70,71].

Prostaglandins are potent vasodilators that have proven to be efficacious in Raynaud's phenomenon. Epoprostenol (prostacyclin) is a vasodilator and potentially provides "protection" to the endothelium. Parenteral administration of its analog, iloprost, improves severe Raynaud's attacks and digital ischemic ulcerations [72]; short infusions of iloprost seem to be as effective in the reduction of number and severity of attacks as daily nifedipine [73]. Iloprost is being used chronically by intermittent intravenous infusion for the treatment of Raynaud's phenomenon and scleroderma with some success [74]. Oral prostacyclin analogs are not yet available or effective for the treatment of Raynaud's phenomenon [75].

Other commonly used vasodilators include nitrates (topical, sublingual, or oral) and α-sympatholytics, such as Prazosin. Although helpful in some patients who cannot tolerate a calcium channel blocker, these agents are of limited value for the long-term management of secondary Raynaud's phenomenon.

Novel vasodilator therapies

Several novel therapies are being used and some formal investigations are underway. These include the use of endothelin inhibitors, nitric oxide substrates (eg, L-arginine), phosphodiesterase inhibitors, selective serotonin reuptake inhibitors, angiotensin II receptor inhibitors, and angiotensin-converting enzyme inhibitors.

Endothelin inhibitors (eg, bosentan) may act as vasodilators and may inhibit smooth muscle activation and proliferation. Recently, there were encouraging reports on the successful therapy of Raynaud's phenomenon and digital ulcers in patients who had scleroderma [76,77]. The effectiveness of bosentan in the prevention of digital ulcers was demonstrated recently in a randomized, prospective, placebo-controlled, double-blind trial that involved 122 patients who had scleroderma [78]. A recent case series reported that bosentan led to complete cessation of Raynaud's symptoms in 4 patients [79]. Interest in the use of sildenafil for the vascular disease of scleroderma also has increased. Although case reports suggest some benefit in Raynaud's phenomenon, no formal clinical trials have been reported to guide its use in MCTD or other similar diseases. Serotonin is a potent vasoconstrictor that is released from nerve endings and during platelet activation. For this reason, selective serotonin reuptake inhibitors are believed to be helpful in the treatment of Raynaud's phenomenon. Fluoxetine (20 mg/d) was compared with nifedipine (40 mg/d) in patients who had primary and secondary Raynaud's phenomenon [80]. In this pilot study, fluoxetine statistically improved the frequency and severity of Raynaud's attacks, whereas the improvement with nifedipine did not reach statistical significance. A positive response was greater in patients who had primary Raynaud's phenomenon than in those who had secondary Raynaud's phenomenon. Its benefit in MCTD has not been tested. Pentoxifylline and cilostazol are reported to improve Raynaud's symptoms [81,82]; however a recent double-blind controlled trial with cilostazol did not show any improvement in symptoms [83].

Although the authors have used each of these novel agents with some success either alone or in combination with the standard calcium channel blocker therapy, they limit their use to complex cases that do not respond to a calcium channel blocker alone. Placebo and weather-controlled trials are needed to better define their role in MCTD.

Ischemia-reperfusion and tissue injury from free radical formation likely is a major cause of vessel and tissue injury in MCTD as is proposed for scleroderma. The use of antioxidants may prevent disease or reduce tissue damage. 3-Hydroxy-3 methylglutaryl-CoA reductase inhibitors (statins) [84] may be beneficial in MCTD-associated vasculopathy because they may reduce platelet aggregation, inhibit vascular smooth muscle proliferation, and improve endothelial dysfunction which promote vasodilatation. The use of statin therapy has not been studied formally and cannot be recommended for routine use; however, patients who have MCTD should be screened for hyperlipidemia and the statins should be used when indicated.

Antiplatelet and anticoagulant therapy

The frequent findings of microthrombi on histology of patients who have MCTD suggest a potential benefit from antiplatelet therapy or anticoagulation. Activated platelets are the source of several key vasospastic substances, such as serotonin and thromboxane A2, and could contribute to the manifestation of Raynaud's phenomenon. Two controlled trials that studied aspirin and dipyridamole in patients who had scleroderma failed to show a significant effect [85,86]. The authors still recommend that patients who have MCTD be placed on antiplatelet therapy with 81 mg of aspirin daily, unless there is a contraindication.

Management of critical digital ischemia

When patients develop larger vessel digit-threatening ischemia, a more aggressive approach is necessary. The authors consider this to be a medical emergency that requires hospitalization. A warm environmental temperature, bed rest to decrease trauma and activity of the involved limb, and appropriate pain control is essential. Vasodilator therapy should be maximized with titration of calcium channel blockers to a full, tolerated dose. Local infiltration of lidocaine or bupivicaine at the base of the involved finger to produce a rapid chemical sympathectomy can improve blood flow and rapidly reduce ischemic pain. This can be given intermittently while waiting for other vasodilator therapy to take full effect.

For patients who have rapidly advancing ischemic tissue, anticoagulant therapy is initiated; although there are no formal studies, the use of heparin for 24 to 72 hours during an acute crisis makes sense. Chronic anticoagulation is not recommended, but also has not been studied. A recent study demonstrated the benefit of low-molecular–weight heparin for symptomatic improvement in primary and secondary Raynaud's phenomenon [87]. In cases of rapidly progressing ischemia that fail to respond to standard vasodilatory therapy, intravenous iloprost, alprostadil, or epoprostenol can be given.

When medical therapy fails, several surgical interventions can be considered. These include proximal or distal (digital) sympathectomy and arterial reconstruction. Distal sympathectomy is associated with a lower complication rate than proximal sympathectomy, but the long-term outcome has not been well-documented [88,89]. As with other vasodilator therapy, sympathectomy is less effective in patients who have secondary Raynaud's phenomenon [90,91].

If there is evidence of larger vessel occlusive disease, such as has been reported at the level of the ulnar or radial arteries, vascular reconstruction can be performed successfully with vein grafts [92]. Therefore, all patients who present with a critical ischemic crisis should have a careful assessment to detect any correctable macrovascular disease. The authors use arterial Doppler studies, magnetic resonance angiography, or angiography to define the magnitude of larger vessel disease in these selected cases.

Digital lesions

Dry skin and subsequent fissures may develop in patients who have MCTD, similar to patients who have systemic sclerosis. The therapeutic approach to these lesions was reviewed recently [93]. Such lesions do not respond well to vasodilatory therapy, and are best taken care of with topical lubricating products (eg, Eucerin, LacHydrin, Vaseline Intensive Care, Theraplex). Wound healing is impaired because of poor circulation, which puts the patient at risk for secondary infections. Therefore, the authors advise patients to take great care to minimize exposure to trauma similar to recommendations for diabetic patients. Active ulcers are treated with soap and water bathing twice daily followed by topical antibiotic ointment and protective dressing. Systemic antibiotic therapy is used for cellulitis or deep secondary infections, including paronychia.

Summary

Raynaud's phenomenon is present almost uniformly in MCTD. Patients who present with Raynaud's phenomenon and a high anti–U1-RNP antibody titer should be watched closely for features of MCTD. In particular, nailfold capillary findings are helpful to distinguish these patients from those who have primary Raynaud's phenomenon. Cardiopulmonary complications, including pulmonary hypertension, are a risk among patients who present with Raynaud's phenomenon and anti–U1-RNP antibodies. Although Raynaud's phenomenon tends to be less severe in patients who have MCTD compared with those who have scleroderma, its pathogenesis seems to be similar. Specific recommendations for therapy for Raynaud's phenomenon in MCTD are not yet established, but it makes sense to follow the management that is used in patients who have scleroderma.

References

[1] Sharp GC, Irvin WS, Tan EM, et al. Mixed connective tissue disease–an apparently distinct rheumatic disease syndrome associated with a specific antibody to an extractable nuclear antigen (ENA). Am J Med 1972;52(2):148–59.

[2] Burdt MA, Hoffman RW, Deutscher SL, et al. Long-term outcome in mixed connective tissue disease: longitudinal clinical and serologic findings. Arthritis Rheum 1999;42(5): 899–909.

[3] Calderon J, Rodriguez-Valverde V, Sanchez Andrade S, et al. Clinical profiles of patients with antibodies to nuclear ribonucleoprotein. Clin Rheumatol 1984;3(4):483–92.

[4] Granier F, Vayssairat M, Priollet P, et al. Nailfold capillary microscopy in mixed connective tissue disease. Comparison with systemic sclerosis and systemic lupus erythematosus. Arthritis Rheum 1986;29(2):189–95.

[5] Bennett RM, O'Connell DJ. Mixed connective tissue disease: a clinicopathologic study of 20 cases. Semin Arthritis Rheum 1980;10(1):25–51.

[6] Jonsson J, Norberg R. Symptomatology and diagnosis in connective tissue disease. II. Evaluations and follow-up examinations in consequence of a speckled antinuclear immuno-fluorescence pattern. Scand J Rheumatol 1978;7(4):229–36.

[7] Alarcon-Segovia D, Villareal M. Classification and diagnostic criteria for mixed connective tissue disease. In: Kasukawa R, Sharp GC, editors. Mixed connective tissue disease and anti-nuclear antibodies. Amsterdam: Elsevier; 1987. p. 33–40.

[8] Gelber AC, Wigley FM, Stallings RY, et al. Symptoms of Raynaud's phenomenon in an inner-city African-American community: prevalence and self-reported cardiovascular comorbidity. J Clin Epidemiol 1999;52(5):441–6.

[9] Block JA, Sequeira W. Raynaud's phenomenon. Lancet 2001;357(9273):2042–8.

[10] Maricq HR, Carpentier PH, Weinrich MC, et al. Geographic variation in the prevalence of Raynaud's phenomenon: Charleston, SC, USA, vs Tarentaise, Savoie, France. J Rheumatol 1993;20(1):70–6.

[11] Estes D, Christian CL. The natural history of systemic lupus erythematosus by prospective analysis. Medicine (Baltimore) 1971;50(2):85–95.

[12] Hochberg MC, Boyd RE, Ahearn JM, et al. Systemic lupus erythematosus: a review of clinico-laboratory features and immunogenetic markers in 150 patients with emphasis on demographic subsets. Medicine (Baltimore) 1985;64(5):285–95.

[13] Garcia-Carrasco M, Siso A, Ramos-Casals M, et al. Raynaud's phenomenon in primary Sjogren's syndrome. Prevalence and clinical characteristics in a series of 320 patients. J Rheumatol 2002;29(4):726–30.

[14] Saraux A, Allain J, Guedes C, et al. Raynaud's phenomenon in rheumatoid arthritis. Br J Rheumatol 1996;35(8):752–4.

[15] De Angelis R, Cerioni A, Del Medico P, et al. Raynaud's phenomenon in undifferentiated connective tissue disease (UCTD). Clin Rheumatol 2005;24(2):145–51.

[16] Mosca M, Neri R, Bencivelli W, et al. Undifferentiated connective tissue disease: analysis of 83 patients with a minimum followup of 5 years. J Rheumatol 2002;29(11):2345–9.

[17] Sharp GC, Irvin WS, May CM, et al. Association of antibodies to ribonucleoprotein and Sm antigens with mixed connective-tissue disease, systematic lupus erythematosus and other rheumatic diseases. N Engl J Med 1976;295(21):1149–54.

[18] Tuffanelli DL, Winkelmann RK. Systemic scleroderma, A clinical study of 727 cases. Arch Dermatol 1961;84:359–71.

[19] Parker MD. Ribonucleoprotein antibodies: frequency and clinical significance in systemic lupus erythematosus, scleroderma, and mixed connective tissue disease. J Lab Clin Med 1973;82(5): 769–75.

[20] Cohen ML, Dawkins B, Dawkins RL, et al. Clinical significance of antibodies to ribo-nucleoprotein. Ann Rheum Dis 1979;38(1):74–8.

[21] Kasukawa R, Tojo T, Miyawaki S. Preliminary diagnostic criteria for classification of mixed

connective tissue disease. In: Kasukawa R, Sharp GC, editors. Mixed connective tissue disease and anti-nuclear antibodies. Amsterdam: Elsevier; 1987. p. 41–7.

[22] Sharp GC. Diagnostic criteria for classification of mixed connective tissue disease. In: Kasukawa R, Sharp GC, editors. Mixed connective tissue disease and anti-nuclear antibodies. Amsterdam: Elsevier; 1987. p. 23–32.

[23] Kahn MF, Appelboom T. Syndrome de Sharp. In: Kahn MF, Peltier AP, Meyer O, et al, editors. Les Maladies Systemiques. Paris: Flammarion; 1991. p. 545–52.

[24] Houtman PM, Kallenberg CG, Fidler V, et al. Diagnostic significance of nailfold capillary patterns in patients with Raynaud's phenomenon. An analysis of patterns discriminating patients with and without connective tissue disease. J Rheumatol 1986;13(3):556–63.

[25] Zufferey P, Depairon M, Chamot AM, et al. Prognostic significance of nailfold capillary microscopy in patients with Raynaud's phenomenon and scleroderma-pattern abnormalities. A six-year follow-up study. Clin Rheumatol 1992;11(4):536–41.

[26] Monticone G, Colonna L, Palermi G, et al. Quantitative nailfold capillary microscopy findings in patients with acrocyanosis compared with patients having systemic sclerosis and control subjects. J Am Acad Dermatol 2000;42(5 Pt 1):787–90.

[27] Maricq HR. Wide-field capillary microscopy. Arthritis Rheum 1981;24(9):1159–65.

[28] Blockmans D, Vermylen J, Bobbaers H. Nailfold capillaroscopy in connective tissue disorders and in Raynaud's phenomenon. Acta Clin Belg 1993;48(1):30–41.

[29] Maricq HR, LeRoy EC, D'Angelo WA, et al. Diagnostic potential of in vivo capillary microscopy in scleroderma and related disorders. Arthritis Rheum 1980;23(2):183–9.

[30] Furtado RN, Pucinelli ML, Cristo VV, et al. Scleroderma-like nailfold capillaroscopic abnormalities are associated with anti-U1-RNP antibodies and Raynaud's phenomenon in SLE patients. Lupus 2002;11(1):35–41.

[31] Lefford F, Edwards JC. Nailfold capillary microscopy in connective tissue disease: a quantitative morphological analysis. Ann Rheum Dis 1986;45(9):741–9.

[32] Hesselstrand R, Scheja A, Shen GQ, et al. The association of antinuclear antibodies with organ involvement and survival in systemic sclerosis. Rheumatology (Oxford) 2003;42(4):534–40.

[33] Mattioli M, Reichlin M. Characterization of a soluble nuclear ribonucleoprotein antigen reactive with SLE sera. J Immunol 1971;107(5):1281–90.

[34] Reichlin M, Mattioli M. Correlation of a precipitin reaction to an RNAprotein antigen and a low prevalence of nephritis in patients with systemic lupus erythematosus. N Engl J Med 1972;286(17):908–11.

[35] Mosca M, Tavoni A, Neri R, et al. Undifferentiated connective tissue diseases: the clinical and serological profiles of 91 patients followed for at least 1 year. Lupus 1998;7(2):95–100.

[36] Danieli MG, Fraticelli P, Franceschini F, et al. Five-year follow-up of 165 Italian patients with undifferentiated connective tissue diseases. Clin Exp Rheumatol 1999;17(5):585–91.

[37] Ihn H, Yamane K, Yazawa N, et al. Distribution and antigen specificity of anti-U1RNP antibodies in patients with systemic sclerosis. Clin Exp Immunol 1999;117(2):383–7.

[38] Kuwana M, Kaburaki J, Okano Y, et al. Clinical and prognostic associations based on serum antinuclear antibodies in Japanese patients with systemic sclerosis. Arthritis Rheum 1994;37(1):75–83.

[39] Hoffman IE, Peene I, Meheus L, et al. Specific antinuclear antibodies are associated with clinical features in systemic lupus erythematosus. Ann Rheum Dis 2004;63(9):1155–8.

[40] ter Borg EJ, Groen H, Horst G, et al. Clinical associations of antiribonucleoprotein antibodies in patients with systemic lupus erythematosus. Semin Arthritis Rheum 1990;20(3):164–73.

[41] Nakano M, Hasegawa H, Takada T, et al. Pulmonary diffusion capacity in patients with systemic lupus erythematosus. Respirology 2002;7(1):45–9.

[42] Pettersson I, Hinterberger M, Mimori T, et al. The structure of mammalian small nuclear ribonucleoproteins. Identification of multiple protein components reactive with anti-(U1)ribonucleoprotein and anti-Sm autoantibodies. J Biol Chem 1984;259(9):5907–14.

[43] Pettersson I, Wang G, Smith EI, et al. The use of immunoblotting and immunoprecipitation of (U) small nuclear ribonucleoproteins in the analysis of sera of patients with mixed connective

tissue disease and systemic lupus erythematosus. A cross-sectional, longitudinal study. Arthritis Rheum 1986;29(8):986–96.

[44] Habets WJ, de Rooij DJ, Salden MH, et al. Antibodies against distinct nuclear matrix proteins are characteristic for mixed connective tissue disease. Clin Exp Immunol 1983;54(1):265–76.

[45] Wigley FM, Wise RA, Miller R, et al. Anticentromere antibody as a predictor of digital ischemic loss in patients with systemic sclerosis. Arthritis Rheum 1992;35(6):688–93.

[46] Schachna L, Wigley FM, Morris S, et al. Recognition of granzyme B-generated autoantigen fragments in scleroderma patients with ischemic digital loss. Arthritis Rheum 2002;46(7): 1873–84.

[47] Flavahan NA, Flavahan S, Liu Q, et al. Increased alpha2-adrenergic constriction of isolated arterioles in diffuse scleroderma. Arthritis Rheum 2000;43(8):1886–90.

[48] Udvardy M, Bodolay E, Szegedi G, et al. Alterations of primary haemostasis in mixed connective tissue disease (MCTD). Thromb Res 1991;63(3):281–6.

[49] Sawai T, Tutikawa K, Watanabe T, et al. [A case of mixed connective tissue disease (MCTD) complicating pulmonary hypertension and portal hypertension]. Ryumachi 1988;28(3):164–9 [in Japanese].

[50] Pallis M, Hopkinson N, Lowe J, et al. An electron microscopic study of muscle capillary wall thickening in systemic lupus erythematosus. Lupus 1994;3(5):401–7.

[51] von Bierbrauer A, Barth P, Willert J, et al. Electron microscopy and capillaroscopically guided nailfold biopsy in connective tissue diseases: detection of ultrastructural changes of the microcirculatory vessels. Br J Rheumatol 1998;37(12):1272–8.

[52] Magro CM, Crowson AN, Regauer S. Mixed connective tissue disease. A clinical, histologic, and immunofluorescence study of eight cases. Am J Dermatopathol 1997;19(3):206–13.

[53] Singsen BH, Swanson VL, Bernstein BH, et al. A histologic evaluation of mixed connective tissue disease in childhood. Am J Med 1980;68(5):710–7.

[54] Sullivan WD, Hurst DJ, Harmon CE, et al. A prospective evaluation emphasizing pulmonary involvement in patients with mixed connective tissue disease. Medicine (Baltimore) 1984; 63(2):92–107.

[55] Braun J, Sieper J, Schwarz A, et al. Widespread vasculopathy with hemolytic uremic syndrome, perimyocarditis and cystic pancreatitis in a young woman with mixed connective tissue disease. Case report and review of the literature. Rheumatol Int 1993;13(1):31–6.

[56] Yamaguchi T, Ohshima S, Tanaka T, et al. Renal crisis due to intimal hyperplasia in a patient with mixed connective tissue disease (MCTD) accompanied by pulmonary hypertension. Intern Med 2001;40(12):1250–3.

[57] de Rooij DJ, Habets WJ, van de Putte LB, et al. Use of recombinant RNP peptides 70K and A in an ELISA for measurement of antibodies in mixed connective tissue disease: a longitudinal follow up of 18 patients. Ann Rheum Dis 1990;49(6):391–5.

[58] Taylor MH, McFadden JA, Bolster MB, et al. Ulnar artery involvement in systemic sclerosis (scleroderma). J Rheumatol 2002;29(1):102–6.

[59] Sgonc R, Gruschwitz MS, Boeck G, et al. Endothelial cell apoptosis in systemic sclerosis is induced by antibody-dependent cell-mediated cytotoxicity via CD95. Arthritis Rheum 2000; 43(11):2550–62.

[60] Bodolay E, Bojan F, Szegedi G, et al. Cytotoxic endothelial cell antibodies in mixed connective tissue disease. Immunol Lett 1989;20(2):163–7.

[61] Bodolay E, Csipo I, Gal I, et al. Anti-endothelial cell antibodies in mixed connective tissue disease: frequency and association with clinical symptoms. Clin Exp Rheumatol 2004;22(4): 409–15.

[62] Okawa-Takatsuji M, Aotsuka S, Uwatoko S, et al. Endothelial cell-binding activity of anti-U1-ribonucleoprotein antibodies in patients with connective tissue diseases. Clin Exp Immunol 2001;126(2):345–54.

[63] Okawa-Takatsuji M, Aotsuka S, Uwatoko S, et al. Increase of cytokine production by pulmonary artery endothelial cells induced by supernatants from monocytes stimulated with autoantibodies against U1-ribonucleoprotein. Clin Exp Rheumatol 1999;17(6):705–12.

[64] Okawa-Takatsuji M, Aotsuka S, Fujinami M, et al. Up-regulation of intercellular adhesion molecule-1 (ICAM-1), endothelial leukocyte adhesion molecule-1 (ELAM-1) and class II MHC molecules on pulmonary artery endothelial cells by antibodies against U1-ribonucleoprotein. Clin Exp Immunol 1999;116(1):174–80.

[65] Okawa-Takatsuji M, Aotsuka S, Uwatoko S, et al. Enhanced synthesis of cytokines by peripheral blood monocytes cultured in the presence of autoantibodies against U1-ribonucleoprotein and/or negatively charged molecules: implication in the pathogenesis of pulmonary hypertension in mixed connective tissue disease (MCTD). Clin Exp Immunol 1994;98(3):427–33.

[66] Weber E, Rossi A, Solito R, et al. Focal adhesion molecules expression and fibrillin deposition by lymphatic and blood vessel endothelial cells in culture. Microvasc Res 2002;64(1):47–55.

[67] Tan FK, Arnett FC, Antohi S, et al. Autoantibodies to the extracellular matrix microfibrillar protein, fibrillin-1, in patients with scleroderma and other connective tissue diseases. J Immunol 1999;163(2):1066–72.

[68] Lundberg I, Antohi S, Takeuki K, et al. Kinetics of anti-fibrillin-1 autoantibodies in MCTD and CREST syndrome. J Autoimmun 2000;14(3):267–74.

[69] Thompson AE, Shea B, Welch V, et al. Calcium-channel blockers for Raynaud's phenomenon in systemic sclerosis. Arthritis Rheum 2001;44(8):1841–7.

[70] Kallenberg CG, Wouda AA, Meems L, et al. Once daily felodipine in patients with primary Raynaud's phenomenon. Eur J Clin Pharmacol 1991;40(3):313–5.

[71] Schmidt JF, Valentin N, Nielsen SL. The clinical effect of felodipine and nifedipine in Raynaud's phenomenon. Eur J Clin Pharmacol 1989;37(2):191–2.

[72] Wigley FM, Seibold JR, Wise RA, et al. Intravenous iloprost treatment of Raynaud's phenomenon and ischemic ulcers secondary to systemic sclerosis. J Rheumatol 1992;19(9):1407–14.

[73] Rademaker M, Cooke ED, Almond NE, et al. Comparison of intravenous infusions of iloprost and oral nifedipine in treatment of Raynaud's phenomenon in patients with systemic sclerosis: a double blind randomised study. BMJ 1989;298(6673):561–4.

[74] Scorza R, Caronni M, Mascagni B, et al. Effects of long-term cyclic iloprost therapy in systemic sclerosis with Raynaud's phenomenon. A randomized, controlled study. Clin Exp Rheumatol 2001;19(5):503–8.

[75] Wigley FM, Korn JH, Csuka ME, et al. Oral iloprost treatment in patients with Raynaud's phenomenon secondary to systemic sclerosis: a multicenter, placebo-controlled, double-blind study. Arthritis Rheum 1998;41(4):670–7.

[76] Black CM, Korn JH, Mayes MD, et al. Improvements in the net ulcer burden and hand functionality in patients with digital ulcers related to systemic sclerosis. Arthritis Rheum 2003;48(Suppl):S454–5.

[77] Humbert M, Cabane J. Successful treatment of systemic sclerosis digital ulcers and pulmonary arterial hypertension with endothelin receptor antagonist bosentan. Rheumatology (Oxford) 2003;42(1):191–3.

[78] Korn JH, Mayes M, Matucci Cerinic M, et al. Digital ulcers in systemic sclerosis: prevention by treatment with bosentan, an oral endothelin receptor antagonist. Arthritis Rheum 2004; 50(12):3985–93.

[79] Ramos-Casals M, Brito-Zeron P, Nardi N, et al. Successful treatment of severe Raynaud's phenomenon with bosentan in four patients with systemic sclerosis. Rheumatology (Oxford) 2004;43(11):1454–6.

[80] Coleiro B, Marshall SE, Denton CP, et al. Treatment of Raynaud's phenomenon with the selective serotonin reuptake inhibitor fluoxetine. Rheumatology (Oxford) 2001;40(9):1038–43.

[81] Goldberg J, Dlesk A. Successful treatment of Raynaud's phenomenon with pentoxifylline. Arthritis Rheum 1986;29(8):1055–6.

[82] Dean SM, Satiani B. Three cases of digital ischemia successfully treated with cilostazol. Vasc Med 2001;6(4):245–8.

[83] Rajagopalan S, Pfenninger D, Somers E, et al. Effects of cilostazol in patients with Raynaud's syndrome. Am J Cardiol 2003;92(11):1310–5.

[84] White CM. Pharmacological effects of HMG CoA reductase inhibitors other than lipoprotein modulation. J Clin Pharmacol 1999;39(2):111–8.

[85] van der Meer J, Wouda AA, Kallenberg CG, et al. A double-blind controlled trial of low dose acetylsalicylic acid and dipyridamole in the treatment of Raynaud's phenomenon. Vasa Suppl 1987;18:71–5.

[86] Beckett VL, Conn DL, Fuster V, et al. Trial of platelet-inhibiting drug in scleroderma. Double-blind study with dipyridamole and aspirin. Arthritis Rheum 1984;27(10):1137–43.

[87] Denton CP, Howell K, Stratton RJ, et al. Long-term low molecular weight heparin therapy for severe Raynaud's phenomenon: a pilot study. Clin Exp Rheumatol 2000;18(4):499–502.

[88] Lowell RC, Gloviczki P, Cherry Jr KJ, et al. Cervicothoracic sympathectomy for Raynaud's syndrome. Int Angiol 1993;12(2):168–72.

[89] Sayers RD, Jenner RE, Barrie WW. Transthoracic endoscopic sympathectomy for hyperhidrosis and Raynaud's phenomenon. Eur J Vasc Surg 1994;8(5):627–31.

[90] Gifford Jr RW, Hines Jr EA, Craig WM. Sympathectomy for Raynaud's phenomenon; follow-up study of 70 women with Raynaud's disease and 54 women with secondary Raynaud's phenomenon. Circulation 1958;17(1):5–13.

[91] Montorsi W, Ghiringhelli C, Annoni F. Indications and results of the surgical treatment in Raynaud's phenomenon. J Cardiovasc Surg (Torino) 1980;21(2):203–10.

[92] Tomaino MM, Goitz RJ, Medsger TA. Surgery for ischemic pain and Raynaud's' phenomenon in scleroderma: a description of treatment protocol and evaluation of results. Microsurgery 2001;21(3):75–9.

[93] Hummers LK, Wigley FM. Management of Raynaud's phenomenon and digital ischemic lesions in scleroderma. Rheum Dis Clin North Am 2003;29(2):293–313.

ELSEVIER
SAUNDERS

RHEUMATIC
DISEASE CLINICS
OF NORTH AMERICA

Rheum Dis Clin N Am 31 (2005) 483–496

Pediatric-Onset Mixed Connective Tissue Disease

Richard J. Mier, MD[a,*], Michael Shishov, MD[b],
Gloria C. Higgins, MD, PhD[c], Robert M. Rennebohm, MD[c],
Dorothy W. Wortmann, MD[d], Rita Jerath, MB, ChB[e],
Ekhlas Alhumoud, MD[f]

[a]Shriners Hospital for Children, 1900 Richmond Road, Lexington, KY 40502, USA
[b]Division of Rheumatology, Cincinnati Children's Hospital Medical Center, 3333 Burnet Avenue,
Cincinnati, OH 45229-3039, USA
[c]Department of Pediatrics, Ohio State University, Childrens Hospital, 700 Childrens Drive,
Columbus, OH, 43205, USA
[d]Department of Pediatrics, Oklahoma University College of Medicine, 4502 East 41st Street,
Tulsa, OK 74135-2512, USA
[e]Department of Pediatrics, Medical College of Georgia, Childrens Medical Center,
Room BG 1016 Dugas Building, Augusta, GA 30912, USA
[f]Department of Allergy and Immunology, McMaster University Medical Center,
1200 Main Street West, HSC, #3V40, Hamilton, Ontario L8N 3Z5, Canada

Reports of pediatric-onset mixed connective tissue disease (MCTD) by Singsen et al [1] and others [2] began appearing within a few years of Sharp et al's [3] 1972 description of adult MCTD. Since then, several reports of pediatric MCTD have appeared that have described in detail the clinical and laboratory circumstances of more than 200 children who have MCTD [4–16].

Despite 30 years of investigation, the place of MCTD in the pantheon of discrete rheumatologic entities continues to be controversial. Enlivening the controversy is the observation that patients who have MCTD—both young and old—exhibit considerable clinical variation cross-sectionally and over time. These inconsistencies or variations in clinical descriptions of children across different reports are a source of confusion regarding pediatric-onset MCTD and may be due to a variety of factors.

Pediatric presentations account for 23% of all cases of MCTD [17]; however, it is a rare disease among children and adolescents and accounted for only 0.6%

* Corresponding author.
E-mail address: rmier@shrinenet.org (R.J. Mier).

0889-857X/05/$ – see front matter © 2005 Elsevier Inc. All rights reserved.
doi:10.1016/j.rdc.2005.04.002   *rheumatic.theclinics.com*

of all pediatric rheumatologic patients in one series [16]. Even in the field of pediatric rheumatology, where uncommon problems are standard, MCTD is rare. Although some of the reported series include large numbers of patients, they often, by necessity, represent compilations of data that are gathered by a large number of clinical observers which introduces the real possibility of observer bias. Among the reports in which patient data are the result of observation and recording by the investigators themselves, the numbers of patients described often are small.

In addition, different investigators have used different criteria for pediatric MCTD which introduces another source of variation. Among nine series of patients who had pediatric-onset MCTD that were published since 1981, four used Kasukawa et al's [18] criteria [10,12–14], one used Sharp's criteria [9], one used Porter's criteria [11], two used no apparent criteria [5,15], and one used all three of the most frequently used criteria [16].

Finally, follow-up periods—important in a disease with manifestations that tend to drift over time—vary considerably from report to report. They may not be short for pediatric follow-up studies but they may not be adequate to know for certain what happens to patients who have pediatric-onset MCTD as they age into their third and fourth decades. Variations in reported clinical manifestations, laboratory evaluation, and prognosis have resulted. For example, Kotajima and colleagues [13] found that systemic lupus erythematosus (SLE)-like features were more common among their pediatric patients who had MCTD than among adult patients. Singsen et al [1] reported that thrombocytopenia and cardiac and renal involvement were seen more frequently in pediatric MCTD as opposed to adult MCTD. Oetgen et al [5] described more sclerodermatous skin changes among their pediatric patients compared with adults. Additionally, although some investigators describe poor outcomes in pediatric MCTD [1,5,16], others describe a more benign process [9,13]. Mortality varies considerably from 29% [1] to 2.8% [13], perhaps as a function of time; the former report was from 1977 and the latter was from 1996.

To reduce variation the authors selected four papers [10,12,13,16] that described patients who had pediatric-onset MCTD; all reports were published since 1993, included data on from 14 to 70 patients each, and used the Kasukawa criteria for diagnosis. Two of the four papers reported adequate mean follow-up of from 5 to 9 years. Data from these four reports have been supplemented by data that were collected recently by the authors from 34 pediatric patients who have MCTD from seven pediatric rheumatology centers. These additional patients all meet Kasukawa's criteria, presented before 16 years of age, and have been followed for a mean of 7.1 years (range, 1.4–18.9 years).

Review of data from four papers [9,11,14,15] that did not meet criteria for inclusion in this review provides similar insights into pediatric-onset MCTD compared with data from papers that did meet our inclusion criteria. Data, such as age at presentation, sex, presenting symptomatology, and physical manifestations (eg, sclerodactyly), were similar between the papers that were used and those that were excluded. There were a few variances, however, with reported frequencies of muscle weakness or evidence for myositis which was more frequent in the reports that were not used than in the reports that were used (74% versus 41%). Laboratory data for antinuclear antibody (ANA) positivity, ribonucleoprotein (RNP) antibody positivity, rheumatoid factor positivity, and double-stranded (ds)DNA antibodies were similar in the reports that were and were not used. Decreased serum complement was found more frequently among the patients from the reports that were not used (32% versus 10%).

Kasukawa's criteria

All of the patient information that was obtained from previously published reports, as well as from our newly collected data set, is from subjects who meet Kasukawa's criteria for the diagnosis of MCTD. Kasukawa's criteria were chosen because they have been applied most frequently to pediatric series and because they are more restrictive—the bar is set higher and requires evidence for more than one collagen vascular disease at diagnosis—which assures greater homogeneity.

Patients must meet all three of the following criteria to be diagnosed with MCTD:

- Raynaud's or swollen fingers or hands or both
- Anti-RNP antibody positivity
- At least one abnormal finding from two or more of the following categories:
  ○ Signs or symptoms of SLE (polyarthritis, facial rash, serositis, lymphadenopathy, leukopenia, thrombocytopenia)
  ○ Signs or symptoms of scleroderma (sclerodactyly, pulmonary fibrosis, vital capacity < 80% of normal, carbon monoxide diffusion < 70% of normal, decreased esophageal motility)
  ○ Signs or symptoms of dermatomyositis (muscle weakness, elevated creatine kinase, EMG abnormalities)

Demographic features

Three of the four published series reported patients by gender [10,12,13]. Eighty-nine of 105 patients (85%) were girls, for a male to female ratio of approximately 1 to 6. Eighty-two percent of our recently collected sample of 34 pediatric patients who had MCTD was girls. Only two of the articles recorded the mean age at onset [10,13]; the weighted mean age for those 84 patients was 12.0 years. Our 34 patients exhibited a younger mean age at onset of 9.5 years. Among our cohort, there was a 1.7-year difference between the age at onset of symptoms and the age at diagnosis of MCTD. The earliest ages at presentation among the three reports [10,12,13] were 4.0 years, 5.2 years, and 5 years. Among our patients, the earliest age at onset was 2 years.

The latest ages at presentation among the pediatric patients that were reported in three papers were 15.9 years, 15.6 years, and 15 years—and in our patients was 15.8 years.. This may be related artificially to the fact that pediatric-onset MCTD was defined as occurring before the 16th birthday or that patients were collected from pediatric rheumatology centers. The mean duration of follow-up for the two papers that included this information was 8.1 years [10,13] and the mean duration of follow-up for our 34 patients was 7.1 years (range 1.4–18.9 years).

Information regarding race was not included in any of the four papers under review, although two papers described children from Japan. Among our 34 patients, 70% were white, 27% were black, and 3% were Hispanic.

Prognosis

Two of the four papers reported mortality of 4 patients during follow-up [13,16] among a total of 103 patients. The other two papers [10,12] did not include information regarding deaths and it was difficult to know whether this was related to data collection or to the fact that no children had died. Only one of the reports that described mortality reported an average duration of follow-up. Using this report [13], the annual disease-specific mortality in pediatric MCTD is estimated to be between 3 and 4 per 1000 patients. This seems to be less than the annual disease-specific mortality for pediatric SLE which has been reported to be between 12 and 23 per 1000 patients [19,20]. Of the four deaths that were described, one was related to fulminant sepsis [16], one was related to possible myocarditis [16], one was caused by "pulmonary involvement" [13], and the fourth was due to cardiac failure [13]. None of the 34 patients in the authors' series died during the mean 7.1 years of follow-up.

Mortality seems to be greater among adults who have MCTD. Eleven of 47 (23.4%) adult patients who had MCTD died during the 15 years mean duration of follow-up; this was equivalent to an annual disease-specific mortality of approximately 15 per 1000 patients in one report [17]. In another report, 35% of 17 patients died over a mean disease duration of 6 years [21]; this is equivalent to an annual mortality of approximately 58 per 1000 patients. Sharp et al's [22] multicenter study reported 4% mortality over 6 years which is equivalent to an annual disease-specific mortality of 7 per 1000 patients; this was similar to the 7.5 deaths/1000 patients/year from Nimelstein et al's [23] study of 22 patients who had MCTD. Sullivan et al [24] reported 12% mortality, or 11 MCTD deaths/ 1000 patients/year among 34 adult patients who had MCTD. Miyawaki and Onodera [25,26] reported survival that was equivalent to an annual disease-specific mortality of 18 per 1000 patients among 45 Japanese patients who had MCTD. Even after excluding the one outrider [21], adult-onset MCTD does seem to carry a greater risk for mortality than pediatric-onset disease.

Data regarding disease activity at most recent follow-up was obtained using the following definitions that were developed by Michels [16]: remission (absence of clinical evidence of active disease on laboratory or physical examination);

favorable outcome (absence of organ involvement, minor residual symptoms or signs [eg, mild sclerodactyly or mild Raynaud's phenomenon]); and unfavorable outcome (any clinically evident organ involvement, disability due to joint malfunction, severe Raynaud's phenomenon, severe vasculitis, or severe adverse drug reaction).

Using the above definitions of disease activity, 3% of our 34 pediatric patients who had MCTD were in remission, 82% exhibited a favorable outcome, and 15% exhibited an unfavorable outcome; 77% were in school or employed. Only Michels [16] provided similar data among the four reports from the literature, and he reported remissions in 6% of his patients. Among an adult cohort of 47 patients—23% of whom had developed disease in childhood—who were followed for a mean of 15 years by Burdt and colleagues [17], 36% were in remission, 26% had improved, 15% had continued active disease, and 23% had died. Apparently this reflects a worse prognosis for death among a cohort of patients who mostly had adult-onset MCTD, but a better prognosis for remission among survivors. It is unclear from these data whether pediatric MCTD is inherently less severe but longer lasting than adult disease or whether the authors simply have not followed their patients long enough.

Little functional data were available from the four published reports. In Michels' series [16], only two of 33 children (6%) "demonstrated symptoms resulting in remarkable limitations in the activities of daily life." Among the authors' 34 patients, 68% had a Steinbrocker score of II which indicates "normal function despite discomfort or limitation of a few joints." Twenty-nine percent had a score of III ("able to perform only a few occupational or self-care duties") and one child (3%) had a score of I ("normal"). None of the authors' patients had a Steinbrocker score of IV ("severely impaired with little or no self-care").

Clinical characteristics at presentation

Knowing what pediatric patients who have MCTD look like at presentation is important. Raynaud's phenomenon was present at disease onset in 70% in Kotajima et al's series [13], in all of Yokota's patients [12], and in only 50% of Tiddens et al's [10] series (weighted mean = 73%). Joint disease affected 36% [13] and 57% [10] at presentation. Swollen fingers or hands at presentation—one of two prerequisites for diagnosis using Kasukawa's criteria—was mentioned only by Kotajima and occurred in only 6% of the patients.

Initially, alternative diagnoses to MCTD were made frequently. In the series of Tiddens et al [10] and Yokota [12], the initial diagnosis was MCTD in 34%, JCA/JRA/JIA (chronic arthritis in children) in 20%, SLE in 14%, and myositis in 9% (all weighted means). The remainder were believed to have acute rheumatic fever, fever of unknown origin, undifferentiated connective tissue disease, or Raynaud's disease [10,12]. None of the patients was believed to have scleroderma at presentation. In the authors' series, 65% were believed to have MCTD initially, 12% were believed to have JCA/JRA/JIA, 12% were believed to have Raynaud's

Table 1
Frequencies of clinical features of pediatric-onset mixed connective tissue disease at presentation and
at most recent follow-up among authors' series of 34 patients

Clinical features of MCTD	At presentation (%)[a]	Most recent follow-up (%)[b]
Arthralgia	91	48
Raynaud's disease	81	88
Fatigue	76	38
Arthritis	74	24
Swelling of hands/fingers	65	19
Muscle enzyme elevations	59	23
Myalgia	42	9
Muscle weakness	34	9
Esophageal dysmotility	25	33
Restrictive lung disease	22	64
Decreased CO diffusion	21	58
Finger ulcers/pitting scars	21	24
Headaches	19	9
Gottron's	18	18
Pulmonary fibrosis on CT	14	100[c]
Telangiectasias	12	15
GERD symptoms	12	30
Vasculitis rash	12	12
Sclerodactyly	12	24

[a] Includes data from 3 months before to 3 months after first contact with patient.
[b] Includes data from 3 months before to 3 months after last contact with patient.
[c] n = 2.

disease, 6% were believed to have SLE, and 3% each were believed to have
scleroderma and polymyositis.

In the authors' cohort of 34 patients, arthralgia (91%), Raynaud's disease
(81%), fatigue (76%), arthritis (74%), and hand swelling (65%) were described at
presentation; these frequencies were greater than have been reported previously.
Typically, these initial manifestations also are found at presentation in adults who
have MCTD [17]. Clinical and laboratory manifestations of muscle inflammation
were present commonly at disease onset among the authors' cohort of patients,
including myalgias in 42%, muscle weakness in 34%, and muscle enzyme
elevations in 59% (Table 1); these are more frequent than described in adults who
had MCTD at the time of diagnosis [17].

Clinical manifestations during disease course

Subsequent to presentation among the authors' 34 patients, arthralgias/arthritis
(94%), Raynaud's disease (94%), fatigue (88%), and hand swelling (68%) continued to be common features. There was a small increase in the number of children who had inflammatory muscle disease (67% of children exhibited abnormal
muscle enzymes at some time during their course); this was more frequent
compared with the weighted mean frequency of 44% for pediatric patients who

had MCTD with muscle inflammation in the four studies [10,12,13,16] that are under review (Table 2).

Symptoms of gastroesophageal reflux disease (GERD) also were common (44%) among the authors' 34 patients, although abnormalities of esophageal motility were documented objectively in only 21%. Among the four reports in the literature, GERD symptoms were present in 24% [10,12,13,16].

Table 2
Rates of clinical features during disease course in patients who had pediatric-onset mixed connective tissue disease

Clinical features of MCTD	Authors' data (%)	Previous reports (%)[a]
Arthralgias	94	NA
Raynaud's disease	94	97 (93–100)
Fatigue	88	NA
Arthritis	82	84 (78–97)
Swollen fingers/hands	68	87 (79–91)
Muscle weakness	47	41 (29–70)
GERD	44	24
Headache	44	36 (only one report [10])
Decreased CO diffusion	42	24 (15–26)
Vasculitis rash	38	50 (only one report [10])
Restrictive lung disease	35	33 (24–64)
Pulmonary fibrosis on CT	30[b]	NA
Finger ulcers/pitting scars	27	NA
Sclerodactyly	26	56 (47–86)
Gottron's	24	9 (9–9)
Esophageal dysmotility	21	7 (7–8)
Lymphadenopathy	21	36 (14–43)
Telangiectasias	18	NA
Alopecia	18	7 (only one report [10])
Dysphagia	18	43 (only one report [10])
Mucosal ulcers	18	13 (only one report [13])
Pericarditis	16	14 (3–28)
Xerostomia/parotid swelling	15	20 (19–20)
APA syndrome[c]	13	NA
Pleuritis	12	12 (10–21)
Heliotrope	9	12 (0–15)
Malar rash	9	NA
Systemic hypertension	8	NA
Discoid lesions	6	6 (only one report [13])
Endocarditis	6	NA
Stroke	4	NA
Aseptic meningitis	4	NA
Xerophthalmia	3	NA
Subcutaneous nodules	3	5 (0–29)

Abbreviations: APA, antiphospholid antibody syndrome; CO, carbon monoxide; GERD, gastro-esophageal reflux disease; NA, not available.

[a] Weighted mean frequencies obtained from four reported series of pediatric MCTD [10,12,13,16] with frequency ranges within parentheses.

[b] Data from 10 selected patients.

[c] IgG or IgM antiphospholipid antibodies plus two clinical manifestations.

Although common, arthritis may not always be severe. Although 97% of Michel's [16] patients had arthritis, it was described as severe in only 6%. This is in contrast with the experience of Tiddens et al [10] who observed cartilage or bony destruction or both in 50% of their patients who had pediatric-onset MCTD.

Pulmonary disease is a major source of morbidity and mortality among adults who have MCTD. Burdt and colleagues [17] reported pulmonary hypertension in 23% of their adult cohort of 47 patients, which is a major cause of mortality. Pulmonary disease was present frequently among pediatric patients as well, although it was more varied in type. Restrictive pulmonary disease (<80% of normal lung volume for age) was found in 35% of 23 patients who were tested from the authors' series over the course of their disease, and in 33% of patients from the literature [10,12,13,16]. Carbon monoxide (CO) diffusion was abnormal (<70% of normal) in 42% of 19 of the authors' patients compared with 24% of those from the literature review [10,12,13,16]. The prevalences of restrictive pulmonary disease and decreased CO diffusion were based on a smaller number of patients than in our total cohort; these patients may have been selected because of symptomatology. Therefore, these frequencies represent maximum rates; the true frequencies may be less. Pulmonary fibrosis was present on 3 of 10 CT scans, that were also presumably performed on a selected subpopulation that was believed to be clinically at risk. Among the 17 patients from the author's study population who had an echocardiogram, only 1 (6%) demonstrated pulmonary hypertension, similar to the 9% who had pulmonary hypertension among Kotajima et al's [13] 70 patients. Twelve percent of the authors' series of 34 patients exhibited pleuritis, the same frequency as among the literature reports; 16% of the authors' patients had pericarditis at some point during their clinical course compared with 14% of patients from the literature [12,13,16].

Although unusual at presentation, a vasculitic rash was found at some time during the disease course in 38% of the authors' cohort of 34 pediatric patients who had MCTD. Other cutaneous findings during the course of disease in the authors' series included Gottron's papules (24%), telangiectasias (18%), alopecia (18%), mucosal ulceration (18%), heliotrope (9%), malar rash (9%), discoid skin lesions (6%), and subcutaneous nodules (3%). Previously published reports [10,12,13,16] described similar frequencies (see Table 2).

In keeping with previous observations that MCTD can drift from a predominantly inflammatory presentation to one that is characterized as scleroderma-like [10], 26% of the authors' patients demonstrated sclerodactyly during their disease course compared with 12% at the time of initial presentation. Similar frequencies for the presence of finger ulcerations were 21% at presentation and 27% subsequently. Fifty-six percent of pediatric patients who had MCTD in the literature [10,12,13,16] exhibited sclerodactyly during their disease course; this was a higher prevalence than in the authors' cohort and a rate that is more similar to adult patients who have MCTD [17].

Renal disease, which is uncommon among adults [17], also is uncommon among pediatric patients who have MCTD. During their disease course only 1 (4%) patient exhibited proteinuria among the authors' series of 34 pediatric patients; only 3 had hematuria (10%). One of the authors' 34 patients underwent renal biopsy which demonstrated World Health Organization class II lupus nephritis. Only 6% of children from the four reports [10,12,13,16] were described as having nephritis.

Although xerostomia/parotid swelling was present in only 15% of the authors' 34 patients and xerophthalmia/keratoconjunctivitis sicca was present in only 3%, symptoms of Sjögren's syndrome were present much more frequently (79%) among the 33 pediatric patients who had MCTD that were reported by Michels [16]. Recurrent parotitis or salivary gland involvement were reported by Tiddens et al [10] and Yokota [12] to be present at approximately the same rate as the authors observed—in 21% and 19% of patients, respectively.

Although headache was common (44%) among the authors' 34 patients, other neurologic manifestations largely were absent. One child had a stroke and one had aseptic meningitis, but no patient had transverse myelitis or a peripheral neuropathy. Among the four reports from the literature, only Kotajima et al [13] reported central nervous system manifestations ("seizures or psychosis") among 13% of his 70 patients.

Changes in clinical features from presentation compared with most recent follow-up

Arthralgia, fatigue, arthritis, swelling of fingers or hands, muscle enzyme elevations, myalgia, and muscle weakness were much less frequent among the authors' population of patients who had pediatric-onset MCTD at last follow-up compared with at presentation. Conversely, the presence of restrictive lung disease and decreased CO diffusion were much more frequent (see Table 1). The authors' experience is similar in several respects to that of Tiddens et al [10], who observed that inflammatory myositis-like manifestations decreased in frequency over time, whereas scleroderma-like manifestations increased in frequency. They also observed a persistence of joint abnormalities, something the authors did not observe. The authors' patients did seem to become more "sclerodermatous" over time, with significant increases in the frequencies of restrictive lung disease and decreased CO diffusion. Although increases in abnormal esophageal motility, GERD symptoms, and sclerodactyly also were observed, these increases were more modest (see Table 1).

Frequency of presentation and courses by rheumatologic category

To obtain a better idea of the relative frequencies of myositis-like, lupuslike, and scleroderma-like presentations and subsequent courses, the frequencies of individual manifestations that were associated with each of these three categories were compared. The presence of arthritis, arthralgia, Raynaud's disease, lymphadenopathy, and hand swelling were excluded because they lacked specificity for categorization.

In the authors' series of 34 patients, manifestations of inflammatory muscle disease (muscle enzyme elevations, muscle weakness, myalgias, Gottron's, and heliotrope rash) were present most often at disease onset; frequencies of individual manifestations varied from 9% to 59% (mean = 32%). The next most frequent panel of manifestations were those associated with systemic sclerosis (sclerodactyly, restrictive pulmonary disease, decreased CO diffusion, decreased esophageal motility, pitting fingertip scars, symptoms of GERD, telangiectasias, dysphagia, and pulmonary hypertension); these occurred at disease onset with frequencies that varied from 0% to 25% (mean = 15%). Least frequent were manifestations that usually were associated with SLE (malar rash, pericarditis, pleuritis, leukopenia, thrombocytopenia, mucosal ulceration, discoid lupus, headache, alopecia, proteinuria, hematuria, decreased complement levels, Smith antibodies, anti-dsDNA antibodies, and evidence for antiphospholipid antibody syndrome); these occurred at disease onset with frequencies that varied from 0% to 19% (mean = 6%).

During the disease course, frequencies for manifestations that are associated with myositis increased to 9% to 67% (mean = 40%), manifestations associated with systemic sclerosis increased to 6% to 44% (mean = 26%), and manifestations associated with SLE increased to 4% to 36% (mean = 18%).

At last follow-up, frequencies for manifestations associated with myositis were 3% to 23% (mean = 12%). Frequencies for manifestations associated with scleroderma were 0–64% (mean = 29%). Frequencies for manifestations associated with SLE were 0-27% (mean = 7%).

Although admittedly a rough calculation, it may be inferred from the above that inflammatory presentations in pediatric MCTD do seem to burn out over time, and that scleroderma-like disease may predominate as disease progresses

Table 3

Ranges of frequencies of panels of disease manifestations among the authors' patients who had pediatric-onset mixed connective tissue disease

Disease manifestation	Presentation (mean)[a] (%)	Course (mean)[b] (%)	Follow-up (mean)[c] (%)
SLE-like[d]	0–19 (6)	4–36 (18)	0–27 (7)
Scleroderma-like[e]	0–25 (15)	6–44 (26)	0–64 (29)
Myositis-like[f]	9–59 (32)	9–67 (40)	3–23 (12)

[a] Includes data from 3 months before to 3 months after first contact with patient.

[b] Frequencies during disease course, subsequent to presentation.

[c] Includes data from 3 months before to 3 months after last contact with patient.

[d] Includes malar rash, pericarditis, pleuritis, leukopenia, thrombocytopenia, mucosal ulceration, discoid lupus, headache, alopecia, proteinuria, hematuria, decreased complement levels, Smith antibodies, anti-dsDNA antibodies, and evidence for antiphospholipid antibody syndrome.

[e] Includes sclerodactyly, restrictive pulmonary disease, decreased CO diffusion, decreased esophageal motility, pitting fingertip scars, symptoms of GERD, telangiectasias, dysphagia, and pulmonary hypertension.

[f] Includes muscle enzyme elevations, muscle weakness, myalgias, Gottron's, and heliotrope rash.

(Table 3). This has been described among pediatric-onset MCTD [10] and adult-onset disease [17,24].

Laboratory data

High-titer antibody positivity against U1RNP, part of the spliceosome particle, is a prerequisite for diagnosis using Kasukawa's criteria [18]. Additionally, the presence of high-titer ANA antibodies that demonstrate a speckled pattern is virtually universal in pediatric-onset MCTD, as it is in adult disease (Table 4). Anti-RNP antibodies were reported to disappear over time in adult patients who were in remission [17]; four of the authors' 34 patients (12%) who initially were anti-RNP positive, were negative at the time of last follow-up visit. Rheumatoid factor was present at some time during disease course in 57% of the authors series, and was present at the same rate among the pediatric-onset patients who were described in the literature review [10,12,13,16]. Autoantibodies against dsDNA were found in 24% of the authors' patients and 37% of the patients from the literature [10,12,13,16]. Smith antibodies were present in 17% of the authors' patients and 11% of the patients from the literature [10,12,13,16].

Sjögren's syndrome A and B (SSA and SSB, respectively) antibody positivity was present in 13% and 14% of the authors' patients, respectively. None of the authors' patients had ScL 70 antibodies, anticentromere antibodies, Jo1 antibodies, or PM/Scl antibodies, although the numbers tested were small.

Thrombocytopenia ($< 100,000/mm^3$) was present during the course of disease in 18% of the authors' patients and 10% of the patients from the literature [10,12,13,16]. Leukopenia ($< 4000/mm^3$) was present during disease course in 36% of the authors' patients and 27% of patients who had pediatric MCTD in the four previously published reports [10,12,13,16]. Thirty percent of the authors'

Table 4

Rates of laboratory features during disease course in patients who had pediatric onset mixed connective tissue disease

Laboratory feature	Authors' data (%)	Previous reports (ranges)[a] (%)
RNP antibodies	100	100
ANA antibodies	100	98 (97–100)
Speckled pattern (ANA)	NA	100
Rheumatoid factor	57	57 (14–81)
dsDNA antibodies	24	37 (21–44)
Smith antibodies	17	11 (0–17)
Platelets $< 100,000/mm^3$	18	10 (6–21)
WBC $< 4000/mm^3$	36	27 (21–30)
C3/C4 decreased	30	10 (only one report [12])
Muscle enzyme elevations	67	44 (24–68)

Abbreviation: WBC, white blood cell.

[a] Weighted mean frequencies obtained from four reported series of pediatric MCTD [10,12,13,16] with frequency ranges within parentheses.

patients exhibited reduced C3 or C4 complement levels or both during their disease course; this was greater than the 10% that was described in Yokota's [12] report of 21 children.

Thrombocytopenia among adult patients who had overlap syndrome and RNP positivity was slightly more common (29%) and leukopenia was slightly less common (24%) [26] when compared with patients who had pediatric-onset MCTD. Rheumatoid factor positivity is approximately as frequent in adults (47%) as it is in children [26]. Smith antibodies were present in 11% of adult patients who had MCTD from one series [17], and was associated with progressive, severe disease.

Treatment

Only Tiddens et al [10] provided quantitative data regarding therapy in their series of pediatric-onset MCTD. Nonsteroidal anti-inflammatory medications were used in 78%, corticosteroids were used in 71%, and hydroxychloroquine was used in 50% of their series of 14 patients. Two patients (14%) were treated with azathioprine. The authors' results are similar; at some time during their disease course, 74% of patients were treated with nonsteroidal anti-inflammatory medications, 82% were treated with corticosteroids (mostly orally), and 50% were treated with hydroxychloroquine. In addition, methotrexate was used in 47%, mycophenolate mofetil was used in 15%, etanercept was used in 15%, azathioprine was used in 9%, cytoxan was used in 6%, cyclosporine was used in 3%, and infliximab was used in 3%. Calcium channel blockers also were used frequently, including nifedipine in 26% and amlodipine in 18%. Several other medications were used, including gastroprotective medications, nutritional supplements, antidepressants, and agents to improve blood flow. Each patient in the authors' series averaged more than eight different medications during the course of their disease; all were not taken at the same time.

Summary

One of the reasons why MCTD remains such an enduring focus must be related to the relish that rheumatologists bring to an apparently insolvable controversy. Although perhaps less a disease than a process, labeling a child with MCTD provides the possibility of a roadmap for the clinician as the child and his or her problems progress, regress, and change.

Pediatric-onset MCTD and adult-onset MCTD look similar, at least in the beginning, with high rates of arthralgia, Raynaud's disease, fatigue, arthritis, and hand swelling. Although not benign, pediatric-onset MCTD carries less mortality than pediatric-onset SLE or adult-onset MCTD, probably because pulmonary hypertension seems to be less of a problem in pediatric MCTD than in adult MCTD, as far as can be determined on the basis of medium-term follow-up studies. From the authors' series, children tend to do well with a favorable outcome 82% of the time, although disease remission is uncommon (3%). Furthermore, patients who have pediatric-onset MCTD do well functionally, as measured by Steinbrocker class. Additionally, 77% are students or are employed.

The most frequent presentation included manifestations that were myositis-like. Like Tiddens and colleagues [10], the authors observed a shift toward scleroderma over time, although not to the same degree that they did.

A lot can be learned from the authors' pediatric patients regarding this elusive concept. Perhaps more useful for clinical decision-making than nosologically satisfying, MCTD as a diagnostic label in children may provide insight as more is learned about HLA associations and autoantibody specificity. Defining clinical outcomes among patients who have pediatric-onset MCTD requires long-term studies of 20 years or more because most of the authors' pediatric patients continue to have active disease and change, even as they graduate from pediatric to adult rheumatology centers.

Acknowledgments

The authors gratefully acknowledge the assistance of J. Kenneth Herd, MD, Professor Emeritus of Pediatrics, East Tennessee State University College of Medicine, Johnson City, Tennessee and Hermine Brunner, MD, Childrens Hospital Medical Center, Cincinnati, Ohio.

References

[1] Singsen BH, Swanson VL, Kornreich HK, et al. Mixed connective tissue disease in childhood: a clinical and serologic survey. J Pediatr 1977;90:893–900.
[2] Fraga A, Gudino J, Ramos-Niembro F, et al. Mixed connective tissue disease in childhood. Am J Dis Child 1978;132:263–5.
[3] Sharp GC, Irvin WS, Tan EM, et al. Mixed connective tissue disease—an apparently distinct rheumatic disease syndrome associated with a specific antibody to an extractable nuclear antigen (ENA). Am J Med 1972;52:148–59.
[4] Singsen BH, Swanson VL, Bernstein BH, et al. A histologic evaluation of mixed connective tissue disease in childhood. Am J Med 1980;68:710–7.
[5] Oetgen WJ, Boice JA, Lawless OJ. Mixed connective tissue disease in children and adolescents. Pediatrics 1981;67:333–7.
[6] Savouret JF, Chudwin DS, Wara DW, et al. Clinical and laboratory findings in childhood mixed connective tissue disease: presence of antibody to ribonucleoprotein containing the small nuclear ribonucleic acid U1. J Pediatr 1983;102:841–6.
[7] Itzkowitch D, Alexander M, Famacy JP, et al. Overlapping connective tissue disease in children. Clin Rheumatol 1983;2:375–80.
[8] Allen RC, St-Cyr C, Maddison PJ, et al. Overlap connective tissue syndromes. Arch Dis Child 1986;61:284–8.
[9] deRooij DJ, Fiselier TH, vandePutte LB, et al. Juvenile-onset mixed connective tissue disease: clinical, serological and follow-up data. Scand J Rheumatol 1989;18:157–60.

[10] Tiddens HAWM, vanderNet JJ, deGraeff-Meeder ER, et al. Juvenile-onset mixed connective
     tissue disease: longitudinal follow-up. J Pediatr 1993;122:191–7.
[11] Hoffman RW, Cassidy JT, Takeda Y, et al. U1–70-kd autoantibody-positive mixed connective
     tissue disease in children: a longitudinal clinical and serologic analysis. Arthritis Rheum 1993;
     36:1599–602.
[12] Yokota S. Mixed connective tissue disease in childhood. Acta Paediatr Jpn 1993;35:472–9.
[13] Kotajima L, Aotsuka S, Sumiya M, et al. Clinical features of patients with juvenile onset mixed
     connective tissue disease: Analysis of data collected in a nationwide collaborative study in Japan.
     J Rheumatol 1996;23:1088–94.
[14] Mier R, Ansell B, Hall MA, et al. Long term follow-up of children with mixed connective tissue
     disease. Lupus 1996;5:221–6.
[15] Yokota S, Imagawa T, Katakura S, et al. Mixed connective tissue disease in childhood:
     a nationwide retrospective study in Japan. Acta Paediatr Jpn 1997;39:273–6.
[16] Michels H. Course of mixed connective tissue disease in children. Ann Med 1997;29:359–64.
[17] Burdt MA, Hoffman RW, Deutscher SL, et al. Long-term outcome in mixed connective tissue
     disease: longitudinal clinical and serologic findings. Arthritis Rheum 1999;42:899–909.
[18] Kasukawa R, Tojo T, Miyawaki S. Preliminary diagnostic criteria for classification of mixed
     connective tissue disease. In: Kasukawa R, Sharp GC, editors. Mixed connective tissue disease
     and antinuclear antibodies. Amsterdam: Elsevier; 1987. p. 41–7.
[19] Wang LC, Yang YH, Lu MY, et al. Retrospective analysis of mortality and morbidity of pediatric
     systemic lupus erythematosus in the past two decades. J Microbial Immunol Infect 2003;36:
     203–8.
[20] Bishnoi A, Barron AC, Graham TB, et al. Long-term outcomes of childhood-onset systemic
     lupus erythematosus (cSLE) [abstract]. Arthritis Rheum 2004;50:S533.
[21] Garcia-de la Torre I, Salazar-Paramo M, Salmon-de la Torre G. Mixed connective tissue disease.
     A clinico-serological study of 17 cases. Mol Biol Rep 1996;23:153–7.
[22] Sharp GC, Irvin WS, May CM, et al. Association of antibodies to ribonucleoprotein and Sm
     antigens with mixed connective-tissue disease, systemic lupus erythematosus and other
     rheumatic diseases. N Engl J Med 1976;295:1149–54.
[23] Nimelstein SH, Brody S, McShane D, et al. Mixed connective tissue disease: a subsequent
     evaluation of the original 25 patients. Medicine (Baltimore) 1980;59:239–48.
[24] Sullivan WD, Hurst DJ, Harmon CE, et al. A prospective evaluation emphasizing pulmonary
     involvement in patients with mixed connective tissue disease. Medicine (Baltimore) 1984;63:
     92–107.
[25] Miyawaki S, Onodera H. Clinical course and prognosis of patients with MCTD. In: Kakusawa R,
     Sharp G, editors. MCTD and antinuclear antibodies. Amsterdam: Excerpta Medica; 1987. p. 331.
[26] Lazaro MA, Cocco JAM, Catoggio LJ, et al. Clinical and serologic characteristics of patients
     with overlap syndrome: is mixed connective tissue disease a distinct clinical entity? Medicine
     1989;68:58–64.

ELSEVIER
SAUNDERS

RHEUMATIC
DISEASE CLINICS
OF NORTH AMERICA

Rheum Dis Clin N Am 31 (2005) 497–508

Pregnancy in Mixed Connective Tissue Disease

Rodanthi C. Kitridou, MD

*Division of Rheumatology and Immunology, Department of Medicine,
University of Southern California Keck School of Medicine,
Los Angeles County–University of Southern California Medical Center, Room 8019,
1200 North State Street, Los Angeles, CA 90033, USA*

Mixed connective tissue disease (MCTD) was described initially by Sharp et al [1] in 1972 as an overlap syndrome with features of lupus, scleroderma, and poly/dermatomyositis (PM/DM) in patients who had antibodies to extractable nuclear antigen and ribonucleoprotein (RNP) specificity. Three more commonly used sets of diagnostic criteria have been proposed for this disease [2–4], all of which have been tested in patients who had systemic lupus erythematosus (SLE), MCTD, scleroderma, PM/DM, and rheumatoid arthritis [5]. Patients who have MCTD may exhibit manifestations of any of the component diseases at different times during the disease course; however, most cases evolve into scleroderma [6]. This article reviews the published experience with pregnancy in MCTD.

Methods

Five papers have addressed pregnancy in MCTD alone, in comparison with, or in addition to, SLE and other systemic rheumatic diseases [7–11]. There are six case reports or letters to the editor about problems with MCTD in pregnancy [12–17], three reports of neonatal lupus in newborns of mothers who had MCTD [18–20], and one study that documented placental changes in two patients who had MCTD [21].

These reports are reviewed, to the extent possible, in terms of maternal disease course during pregnancy and the postpartum period, fetal morbidity and mortality, and therapeutic interventions. The obstetric terms that are used merit definition (Table 1). The data from the above papers are summarized in Table 2.

E-mail address: kitridou@usc.edu

doi:10.1016/j.rdc.2005.04.001   *rheumatic.theclinics.com*

Table 1
Obstetric terms

Term	Definition
Fertility rate	The average number of pregnancies per pregnant patient or control subject
Parity rate	The average number of viable infants per pregnant woman
Adjusted fertility rate	Allows correction for years at-risk for pregnancy (10-year intervals) [8]
Success rate or success percentage	The percentage of viable infants per group of patients (live births per total pregnancies multiplied by 100) [8]. Success percentage allows the evaluation of parity in relationship to fertility.
Spontaneous abortion	The spontaneous termination of pregnancy before 20 weeks' gestation
Still birth or intrauterine fetal death	The spontaneous termination after 20 weeks' gestation
Elective or induced ("therapeutic") abortion	The voluntarily induced termination of pregnancy
Fetal loss	The sum of spontaneous abortions and stillbirths
Total fetal loss	The sum of abortions, stillbirths (IUFDs), and perinatal deaths
Neonatal death	The death of a newborn within 30 days of birth
Perinatal mortality	The sum of stillbirths and neonatal deaths
Recurrent fetal loss or recurrent spontaneous (habitual) abortion	Three or more [22,23], or two or more consecutive spontaneous abortions or intrauterine fetal deaths [24]
Premature (preterm) rupture of membranes	The spontaneous rupture of membranes (amniorrhexis) before the onset of labor and before 37 weeks' gestation
Intrauterine growth restriction	Newborn weight below the 10th percentile for gestational age. Synonyms: small newborn for gestational age, intrauterine malnutrition
Premature or preterm birth	The spontaneous termination of pregnancy with a live birth between 21 and 37 weeks' of gestation
Full-term or term birth	The spontaneous termination of pregnancy with a live birth between 38 and 40 weeks' gestation
Pregnancy-induced hypertension (PIH)	The presence of blood pressure $\geq$ 140/90 mm Hg on at least two occasions, 6 or more hours apart, during the second half of pregnancy in a previously normotensive woman [25]
Preeclampsia	PIH with proteinuria of > 0.3 g/L in the absence of urinary tract infection, or abrupt onset of hypertension and proteinuria after 24 weeks' gestation [26,27]
Severe preeclampsia	Characterized by one or more of the following: blood pressure of $\geq$ 160 mm Hg systolic, or 110 mm Hg diastolic on two readings 6 hours apart, proteinuria > 5 g/24 h, oliguria (<400 mL/24 h), cerebral or visual disturbances, pulmonary edema, or cyanosis
HELLP syndrome	A variant of severe preeclampsia characterized by hemolysis, elevated liver enzymes and low platelets, in addition to the above characteristics [28]
Eclampsia	Severe preeclampsia with malignant hypertension, seizures, and renal failure
Infertility	The lack of conception after 1 year of frequent coitus without contraception

Table 2
Pregnancy in mixed connective tissue disease

First author, year [Ref.]	Patients (N)	Pregnancies[a] (N)	Flares (%)	PIH/Preeclampsia (%)	SAb/IUFD (%)	LB (%)	Premature/IUGR (%)
Bennett et al, 1980 [7]	18	47	0	0	4.3/0	80.9	NR
Kaufman et al, 1982 [8]	22	88 before	NA	0	13.6/3.4	83.0	NR
	10	13 after onset	50% in those with MCTD onset during pregnancy; 30% in those with pre-existing MCTD	5.9	46.2/23.0	30.8	NR
Siamopoulou-Mavridou et al, 1988 [9]	7	19 before onset	NA	0	16/0	84	0
Lundberg et al, 1991 [10]	4	17 before	NA	0	11.8/0	88.2	0
	7	14 after onset	Onset 14.3 35.7[b]	14.3	21.4/0	78.6	0/14.3 CS
Kari, 2001 [11]	5	5	0	0	0	100	20
Selby et al, 1982 [12]	1	1	Yes	No	No	Yes	Yes, CS/NR
Snyder et al, 1985 [13]	1	2	Yes	No	1/0	Yes	No/IUGR, CS
Watanabe et al, 1995 [14]	1	1	Possibly-PHT	No	No	Yes	NR[c]
Yamaguchi et al, 2001 [15]	1	1	Yes-PHT-renal crisis	Renal crisis	No	Yes	CS
Aoki et al, 2001 [16]	1	1	Yes	No	IUFD	No	NA
Horita et al, 2001 [17]	1	2	No, Prednisone Rx	No	No	Yes	No
Nolan et al, 1979 [18]	1	1 CHB, cutaneous NLE, pericarditis	No	No	No	Yes	Yes
Cimaz et al, 2002 [19]	1	1 cutaneous NLE	No	No	No	Yes	No
Fujiwaki et al, 2003 [20]		1 cutaneous NLE	No, Rx 7.5 mg/d prednisolone	No	No	Yes	No/Yes

Abbreviations: CHB, complete heart block; CS, cesarean section; IUFD, intrauterine fetal death; IUGR, intrauterine growth restriction; LB, live birth; NA, not applicable; NLE, neonatal lupus erythematosus; NR, not reported; PHT, pulmonary hypertension; PIH, pregnancy-induced hypertension; SAb, spontaneous abortion.

[a] Pregnancies excluding elective abortions.

[b] Events that may be pregnancy-related or mimic/represent flares. See text.

[c] NR in abstract; article in Japanese.

Results

Full papers

In 1980, Bennett and O'Connell [7] reported a retrospective study of 20 patients who had MCTD. Eighteen had 47 pregnancies that resulted in 38 live births (81% of total pregnancies); 23 pregnancies were uneventful. Two first-trimester miscarriages occurred. These data are well within the data for the general population. Four of the patients had biopsy-proven immune complex nephropathy. There were no toxemias, stillbirths, or postpartum flares reported. Seven pregnancies, however, were unaccounted for.

Two years later, we reported a retrospective study of 31 patients who had MCTD and their pregnancy experience, as compared with 31 patients who had SLE and 51 obstetric controls [8]. At the time of the study, the mean age of the patients who had MCTD was 39.7 years, with a range of 22 to 66 years. Patients who had lupus were younger (mean, 31.9 years; range, 19–60 years), and the healthy controls were even younger (mean, 23.6 years; range 15–40 years). Pregnancy data were divided into "before" and "after" disease onset, as was done commonly at the time.

Fetal outcome

Twenty-two of 31 patients who had MCTD had 96 pregnancies before disease onset, and 10 patients had 17 pregnancies after disease onset. The fertility rate of 4.4 and 1.7, respectively, became 2.5 and 2.4 when adjusted for decades at risk for pregnancy. The control population had a similar adjusted fertility rate of 3.1. Therefore, it seems that fertility was normal in these patients who had MCTD. Of the 96 pregnancies before MCTD onset, 8 were terminated electively. Of the 88 remaining pregnancies, 12 ended with spontaneous abortion (13.6%) and 3 ended with intrauterine fetal death (IUFD; 3.4%), for a fetal loss of 17.0%, and live births (success rate) of 83%. Healthy controls had a fetal loss of 8.3%, which was accounted for entirely by spontaneous abortions. After MCTD onset there was increased fetal loss. Of the 17 pregnancies after MCTD onset, 4 were terminated electively, 6 ended in spontaneous abortion (46.2%), and 3 ended in IUFD (23.0%), for a fetal loss of 69.2%, and live births of 30.8%. The difference in fetal loss after MCTD onset compared with controls, or in MCTD before disease onset was statistically significant.

Maternal morbidity included disease onset during pregnancy in 5 of 10 patients (50%) and disease flares in 3 more patients (30%). The disease onset and flare features included myositis; synovitis; vasculitis; serositis (pleuritis, pericarditis); alopecia; rash; thrombocytopenia; and worsening renal function with increased proteinuria, with or without increased serum creatinine. One patient developed preeclampsia (hypertension and edema), which at the time was considered to be unrelated to MCTD; however, given the similarities between MCTD and SLE in these patients, this may not have been an unrelated complication. These patients were treated with corticosteroid doses that were commensurate with their disease severity. At that time, antimalarial and immunosuppressive therapy was withheld routinely during pregnancy.

A large retrospective study of pregnancy outcomes before the onset of auto-immune rheumatic diseases included 7 patients who had MCTD among 154 patients with 390 pregnancies [9]. This study showed no difference in fetal loss in the patients, compared with 267 pregnancies of 98 healthy control women. There were 19 pregnancies in women before onset of MCTD, with 16 full-term births (84%), 3 spontaneous abortions (16%), and no stillbirths.

Another retrospective study evaluated 20 women who had high anti-RNP antibody titer, 16 of whom had a total of 40 pregnancies [10]. Thirteen of the patients had MCTD, 2 had undifferentiated connective tissue disease (UCTD), and 1 had Sjögren's syndrome. Only the patients who had MCTD are considered here. Four of the 13 patients who had MCTD had 17 pregnancies before disease onset, with 15 ending in full-term deliveries (88.2%), and two spontaneous abortions (11.8%). Of 7 patients with 14 pregnancies after disease onset, one patient had her MCTD onset during pregnancy; there were three spontaneous abortions (21.4%), and 11 full-term deliveries (78.6%). In these 14 pregnancies there was transient proteinuria in 3 patients (21.4%), transient thrombocytopenia in 2 patients (14.3%), deep vein thrombosis in 1 patient (7.1%), and preeclampsia that required cesarean section in 2 pregnancies of 1 patient (14.3%). Another woman had fetal malposition that required cesarean section in both of her pregnancies. In all, there were 5 (35.7%) complications that may be seen in pregnancy, but may appear similar to disease flares. The investigators concluded that all of the observed complications can occur in normal pregnancies, and that the risk of fetal loss and maternal worsening seems slight in such patients.

A study of 30 pregnancies in 30 patients who had a variety of systemic rheumatic diseases included 5 patients who had MCTD [11]. One delivery was premature and no maternal morbidity was reported.

Case reports

Selby et al [12] reported a patient who had MCTD and developed a severe flare 2 days after cesarean section. The flare consisted of fever, pleuritis, myositis, moderately severe restrictive lung disease, diffuse sclerodermatous change, and esophageal hypomotility, all of which improved with high-dose steroid therapy. Delivery was by cesarean section at 33 weeks' gestation because of premature rupture of membranes, and placenta previa with abruption. Her infant girl was healthy.

Snyder et al [13] reported a woman who had Raynaud phenomena, arthritis, leukopenia, and positive antinuclear antibody (ANA) with anti-RNP specificity whose infant—delivered by cesarean section because of fetal distress—had intra-uterine growth restriction (IUGR). The mother had prolonged fever and arthritis during the pregnancy, which was identified as an MCTD flare by her physicians.

Watanabe et al [14] reported a woman who had MCTD who developed acute thromboembolism 2 days post partum and subsequent pulmonary hypertension.

Despite anticoagulation and a moderate pulmonary arterial hypertension (mean pulmonary artery pressure, 45 mm Hg), the patient developed cardiomegaly, shortness of breath with decreased exercise tolerance, and died of right cardiac failure 8 months after delivery. One wonders whether the patient also had myocarditis or myocardiopathy that was due to MCTD flare.

Yamaguchi et al [15] reported a patient who had MCTD and marked pulmonary hypertension who developed renal crisis after a cesarean section delivery. Aggressive therapy with intravenous corticosteroid pulse and intravenous cyclophosphamide reversed the renal crisis. Renal biopsy demonstrated severe intimal hyperplasia without glomerular changes. This is consistent with our study of renal involvement in MCTD; we found arteriolosclerosis in 5 of 12 renal biopsies and severe subintimal sclerosis of arcuate arteries at autopsy in a sixth patient [29].

Aoki et al [16] reported a woman who had MCTD that was in remission and autoimmune hepatitis, which flared after an IUFD in the second trimester of her pregnancy. A liver biopsy showed chronic active hepatitis; antismooth muscle antibody was positive and hepatitis B and C serology was negative. Apparently, only five other patients who had MCTD were reported to have autoimmune hepatitis.

Horita et al [17] reported a patient who had MCTD and nephrotic syndrome that was due to membranous and mesangial nephropathy that responded to steroid therapy. During the patient's two pregnancies the investigators elected to treat her with 10 mg of prednisone per day; the dosage was increased to 30 mg/d during the postpartum period to prevent recurrence of proteinuria. Both neonates were born at term (week 39) without any problems.

Three reports have addressed neonatal lupus erythematosus (NLE) in children of patients who had MCTD (18–20). In 1979, Nolan et al [18] reported complete congenital heart block in the neonate of a patient who had MCTD. The female baby was born prematurely at 32 weeks of gestation, and had complete congenital heart block and a positive ANA with speckled pattern, which later was shown to be anti-RNP. Anti-Ro/SSA (Sjögren's syndrome antigen A) and anti-La/SSB (Sjögren's syndrome antigen B) were not tested for at this early time. The ANA titers gradually decreased from 1:640 to 1:20 from birth to 5 months; this suggested transplacental passage of maternal antibody. At 2 months she developed a severe, scaly, erythematous facial and upper extremity rash with atrophic macules, telangiectasiae, and violaceous upper eyelids. At 4 months she developed pericarditis with cardiac tamponade and sterile pericardial fluid. She had tachypnea with rales, rhonchi, wheezes, and hepatomegaly, all of which improved or resolved with pericardiocentesis. The fluid reaccumulated and she was treated with pericardial window. Her creatine kinase was 190 mIU/mL (upper normal for age is 90 mIU/mL). Her rash was nearly resolved at 7 months and her ANA titer decreased over 5 months.

Cimaz et al [19] reported cutaneous NLE in the newborn of a patient who had MCTD. The baby girl was born at full term (38 weeks) after an uncomplicated pregnancy. There was only anti-RNP in maternal and neonatal serum. Contrary to the usual appearance of cutaneous NLE after the neonate's exposure to ultraviolet light, this newborn was born with an erythematous, depressed, atrophic facial rash that was, in part, scarring that gave the appearance of discoid lupus and suggested in utero occurrence. She also had periungual erythema without vasculitis. She had a positive ANA at 1:320 with anti-RNP specificity. Biopsy of the rash showed a dense lichenoid infiltration with vacuoles at the interface, thinned epidermis, follicular plugging, and mucin deposition. Immunofluorescence study showed scant IgM deposits in the dermo-epidermal junction. No treatment was given and no new lesions appeared in the following months. The investigators pointed out that ultraviolet light exposure was not necessary for the development of cutaneous NLE.

Fujiwaki et al [20] reported a patient who had MCTD who gave birth to a full-term, small for gestational age boy who had cutaneous NLE at 26 days of age. Erythematous papules evolved into a discoid lupus rash with hyperpigmentation that affected the face, trunk, and extended to the inguinal regions and legs. The infant had positive ANA and anti-RNP tests in decreasing titers, from 1:640 and 1:16 to 1:40 and 1:4, respectively, by 6 months of age. Rheumatoid factor, anti-Ro/SSA, anti-La/SSB, anticardiolipin, and lupus anticoagulant antibodies were negative. A biopsy of the rash at 2 months showed atrophic epidermis; mild liquefaction-degeneration of the basal stratum; and dermo-epidermal deposits of IgA, IgM, IgG, C3, and C4 which was consistent with NLE. The gradual decrease of the ANA titers over time is consistent with transplacental passage of maternal antibodies.

Ackerman et al [21] examined placental tissue from nine patients who had systemic rheumatic diseases and adverse fetal outcomes with five losses before 20 weeks of gestation, three stillbirths, and one neonatal death. Six patients had SLE, one had rheumatoid arthritis, and two had MCTD. All patients except those who had MCTD had anticardiolipin or lupus anticoagulant antibodies. One patient who had MCTD had fetal loss at 16 weeks' gestation and the other had a premature infant at 35 weeks' gestation with neonatal death. Both were small for gestational age. Both placentae were small, firm, and fibrotic and showed markedly increased intervillous and perivillous fibrin deposition on light microscopy. The aborted placenta had small infarcts, with deposits of fibrinogen and C3 by immunofluorescence staining. The placenta from the neonatal death showed fibrinogen, IgG, and IgM deposits in the trophoblast basement membrane.

Discussion

Retrospective studies and case reports, although valuable, do not answer definitively the questions about fetal and maternal morbidity in MCTD. Potential reasons for the lack of prospective, controlled studies include the low prevalence of MCTD (in our clinics the ratio of MCTD:SLE is ~1:10), the fact that diagnosis or disease onset of MCTD occurs at a later age, and inherent difficulties in

MCTD diagnosis. Often, MCTD evolves over a period of many years and often is preceded by isolated Raynaud phenomenon, and sometimes is accompanied by swollen hands or sclerodactyly and little else. Many patients who have MCTD are labeled as having UCTD; by the time a more complete clinical picture of MCTD emerges, they may be past their childbearing years. This was true of most of our patients. Another potential confusing factor is that the clinical phenotype of the disease can evolve over time; at times it resembles more one or the other of the component diseases.

Certain useful conclusions may be drawn from the previous studies. First, patients who have MCTD seem to have normal fertility. Second, five of our patients and one of the patients in the Swedish study had onset of MCTD during pregnancy [8,10]. Awareness of this possibility by the rheumatologist and obstetrician/perinatologist will allow prompt recognition and diagnosis of MCTD, and prompt administration of necessary treatment. Third, among our patients and in four of the case reports there were maternal disease flares [8,12,14–16]. Certain events that may accompany pregnancy also may be the expression of disease flares, as in the Swedish patients who had transient proteinuria and transient thrombocytopenia [10]. The investigators considered these events as being caused by the pregnancy. Pregnancy-induced hypertension and preeclampsia occurred in one of our patients [8], in both pregnancies of a patient of Lundberg and Hedfors [10], and renal crisis developed post partum in one of the case reports [15]. Preeclampsia has been linked to the presence of antiphospholipid antibodies (APL) [30–32]. Several of the MCTD studies, including ours, were completed before antiphospholipid testing became a routine practice in SLE and related illnesses. In the recent study by Kari [11], positive APL seemed to occur only in patients who had SLE; in the placental study, the two patients who had MCTD were negative for APL [21]. Preeclampsia in MCTD, however, may be related to vascular changes, such as occur in the glomerulus—notably, arteriolosclerosis and intimal thickening—a finding that was shown in MCTD kidney vessels by us [29], and was seen in the case report by Yamaguchi et al [15]. These changes are akin to scleroderma vascular abnormalities and are believed to underlie the mechanism of hypertension, and perhaps renal crisis, in scleroderma and MCTD.

Fourth, fetal outcome in patients who have MCTD has been favorable, with the exception of our study [8]. Our proportion of only 30.8% live births after MCTD onset is in contrast to the other studies, with live births ranging from 78.6% to 100% [7,10,11]. Some of the reasons for this discrepancy may be that our patients are of an underprivileged socioeconomic level, and may not adhere as well to prenatal care. Our normal controls, however, are derived from the same patient population and had a 91.7% rate of live births. Another reason may be the small size of the patient sample after MCTD onset. There were occasional reports of prematurity [12,18] and IUGR [13,20].

Fifth, apparently neonatal lupus can occur in MCTD although it seems unusual. In one report, an infant who had congenital heart block and cutaneous NLE also had pericarditis, which belies a more severe form of NLE [18]. The mother and child were not tested for anti-Ro/SSA and anti-La/SSB, which have been incriminated in the pathogenesis of CHB [33]. To our knowledge this is the only report of congenital heart block in association with anti-RNP. At the time of the report (1979) anti-Ro/SSA and anti-La/SSB were not obtained routinely. NLE in association with maternal anti–U1-RNP antibodies, in the absence of anti-Ro/SSA and anti-La/SSB, has been reported in a total of 11 infants [34–41]. The cutaneous form of NLE was most prevalent and was seen in 10 of the 11 infants; 1 infant also had transient myasthenia gravis [36] and 1 had thrombocytopenia [41]. Maternal diagnoses ranged from asymptomatic to SLE. The pathogenetic mechanism of NLE related to anti-RNP antibodies has not been elucidated, whereas that related to anti-Ro and anti-La is well-understood, given the presence of the respective antigens in keratinocytes and cardiac cells [42,43].

Sixth and finally, pregnant patients who have MCTD may do well through pregnancy and post partum; however, in view of the sporadic problems with mother and fetus that were mentioned above, and because one of the component diseases is SLE, we recommend the following care guidelines for pregnancy [44]:

Patients who have MCTD should:

- Plan their pregnancy after a time of disease quiescence (eg, at least 5–6 months)
- Have prenatal care by a high-risk obstetrician (perinatologist), with frequent ultrasound evaluations of the fetus, and fetal electrocardiogram as indicated
- Have follow-up by a rheumatologist every month or more frequently
- Have laboratory tests at the onset of pregnancy:
  - Complete blood cell count (repeat every month or as needed)
  - Sedimentation rate (repeat every month or as needed)
  - Chemistry profile (repeat every month or as needed)
  - Urinalysis with microscopic exam (repeat every month or as needed)
  - Anti-RNP
  - Anti-Ro/SSA
  - Anti-La/SSB
  - Anticardiolipin antibodies
  - Lupus anticoagulant
- Have any increase in blood pressure treated promptly by labetalol, α-methyldopa, or nifedipine, the C class antihypertensives that are mostly safe in pregnancy. Patients who had previous renal disease have a 41% chance of developing hypertension during pregnancy and a higher probability of pregnancy-induced hypertension/preeclampsia.
- Have any disease flare treated promptly with corticosteroids
- Be given hydroxychloroquine and azathioprine for MCTD control if needed during pregnancy. The latter's dosage should be decreased by 25% to 50% during the last trimester, to avoid hypogammaglobulinemia in the newborn [44].
- Be given stress-dose corticosteroids during delivery if they are currently being treated with corticosteroids, or took steroids up to 2 years before delivery, Typically, this requires hydrocortisone, 100 mg intravenously, at

the start of the delivery, which is repeated every 8 hours that day. The patient's oral dose may be resumed on the following day.

- Have a neonatologist available at delivery for the (even remote) possibility of congenital heart block, or in the case of prematurity
- Be informed that in the event of fetal distress, maternal renal crisis, or pulmonary hypertension, a cesarean section may be required
- Be considered for treatment with fluorinated steroids (β- or dexamethasone) to promote in utero lung maturation in the event of fetal prematurity
- Have regular postnatal care during the 2 months following delivery.
- Be allowed to breastfeed with maternal prednisone dosages of up to 30 mg/d, antimalarials, and with short-acting nonsteroidal anti-inflammatory drugs. Breastfeeding is not recommended if the mother requires cytotoxic drugs.

Summary

MCTD pregnancy has a modest risk of maternal flare, including preeclampsia, renal crisis, and pulmonary hypertension. Fetal loss was high in our early study, whereas later studies have shown a better fetal outcome. Prematurity, IUGR, and neonatal lupus are uncommon. Overall, the outlook for pregnancy in patients who have MCTD seems to be favorable, as long as the treating rheumatologist and perinatologist are aware of potential problems and are ready to treat them decisively.

References

[1] Sharp GC, Irvin WS, Tan EM, et al. Mixed connective tissue disease—an apparently distinct rheumatic disease syndrome associated with a specific antibody to an extractable nuclear antigen (ENA). Am J Med 1972;52:148–59.
[2] Sharp GC. Diagnostic criteria for classification of MCTD. In: Kasukawa R, Sharp GC, editors. Mixed connective tissue diseases and anti-nuclear antibodies. Amsterdam: Elsevier; 1987. p. 23–32.
[3] Alarcon-Segovia D, Villareal M. Classification and diagnostic criteria for mixed connective tissue diseases. In: Kasukawa R, Sharp GC, editors. Mixed connective tissue diseases and anti-nuclear antibodies. Amsterdam: Elsevier; 1987. p. 33–40.
[4] Kasukawa R, Tojo T, Miyawaki S, et al. Preliminary diagnostic criteria for classification of mixed connective tissue disease. In: Kasukawa R, Sharp GC, editors. Mixed connective tissue diseases and anti-nuclear antibodies. Amsterdam: Elsevier; 1987. p. 41–7.
[5] Alarcon-Segovia D, Cardiel MH. Comparison between 3 diagnostic criteria for mixed connective tissue disease. Study of 593 patients. J Rheumatol 1989;16(3):328–34.
[6] Nimelstein SH, Brody S, McShane D, et al. Mixed connective tissue disease: a subsequent evaluation of the original 25 patients. Medicine 1980;59(4):239–48.
[7] Bennett RM, O'Connell DJ. Mixed connective tissue disease: a clinicopathologic study of 20 cases. Semin Arthritis Rheum 1980;10(1):25–51.
[8] Kaufman RL, Kitridou RC. Pregnancy in mixed connective tissue disease: comparison with systemic lupus erythematosus. J Rheumatol 1982;9:549–55.

[9] Siamopoulou-Mavridou A, Manoussakis MN, Mavridis AK, et al. Outcome of pregnancy in patients with autoimmune rheumatic disease before the disease onset. Ann Rheum Dis 1988; 47(12):982–7.

[10] Lundberg I, Hedfors E. Pregnancy outcome in patients with high titer anti-RNP antibodies. A retrospective study of 40 pregnancies. J Rheumatol 1991;18(3):359–62.

[11] Kari JA. Pregnancy outcome in connective tissue disease. Saudi Med J 2001;22(7):590–4.

[12] Selby C, Richfield M, Croft S, et al. Postpartum flare in mixed connective tissue disease. J Rheumatol 1982;9(2):332–4.

[13] Snyder JM, De Masi AD, Belsky DH. Mixed connective tissue disease in pregnancy: report of a case. J Am Osteopath Assoc 1985;85(1):33–6.

[14] Watanabe R, Tatsumi K, Uchiyama T, et al. Puerperal secondary pulmonary hypertension in a patient with mixed connective tissue disease. Nohon Kyobu Shikkan Gakkai Zasshi 1995;33(8): 883–7.

[15] Yamaguchi T, Ohshima S, Tanaka T, et al. Renal crisis due to intimal hyperplasia in a patient with mixed connective tissue disease (MCTD) accompanied by pulmonary hypertension. Intern Med 2001;40(12):1250–3.

[16] Aoki S, Tada Y, Ohta A, et al. Autoimmune hepatitis associated with mixed connective tissue disease: report of a case and a review of the literature. Nihon Rinsho Meneki Gakkai Kaishi 2001;24(2):75–80.

[17] Horita Y, Tsunoda S, Inenaga T, et al. Pregnancy outcome in nephrotic syndrome with mixed connective tissue disease. Nephron 2001;89(3):354–6.

[18] Nolan RJ, Shulman ST, Victorica BE. Congenital complete heart block associated with maternal mixed connective tissue disease. J Pediatr 1979;95(3):420–2.

[19] Cimaz R, Biggioggero M, Catelli L, et al. Ultraviolet light exposure is not a requirement for the development of cutaneous neonatal lupus. Lupus 2002;11(4):257–60.

[20] Fujiwaki T, Urashima R, Urushidani Y, et al. Neonatal lupus erythematosus associated with maternal mixed connective tissue disease. Pediatr Int 2003;45(2):210–3.

[21] Ackerman J, Gonzalez EF, Gilbert-Barness E. Immunological studies of the placenta in maternal connective tissue disease. Pediatr Dev Pathol 1999;2(1):19–24.

[22] Creagh MD, Malia RG, Cooper SM, et al. Screening for lupus anticoagulant and anticardiolipin antibodies in women with fetal loss. J Clin Pathol 1991;44:45–7.

[23] Mintz G, Niz J, Gutierrez G, et al. Prospective study of pregnancy in systemic lupus erythematosus. Results of a multidisciplinary approach. J Rheumatol 1986;13:732–9.

[24] Love PE, Santoro SA. Antiphospholipid antibodies: anticardiolipin and the lupus anticoagulant in systemic lupus erythematosus (SLE) and in non-SLE disorders. Prevalence and clinical significance. Ann Intern Med 1990;112:682–98.

[25] Wallenburg HCS, Makovitz JW, Dekker GA, et al. Low-dose aspirin prevents pregnancy-induced hypertension and preeclampsia in angiotensin-sensitive primigravidae. Lancet 1986; 1:13.

[26] Brown MA, de Swiet M. Classification of hypertension in pregnancy. Best Pract Res Clin Obstet Gynecol 1999;13:27–39.

[27] Broughton Pipkin F, Roberts JM. Hypertension in pregnancy. J Hum Hypertens 2000;14: 705–24.

[28] Weinstein L. Syndrome of hemolysis, elevated liver enzymes, and low platelet count: a severe consequence of hypertension in pregnancy. Am J Obstet Gynecol 1982;142:159–67.

[29] Kitridou RC, Akmal M, Turkel SB, et al. Renal involvement in mixed connective tissue disease: a longitudinal clinicopathologic study. Semin Arthritis Rheum 1986;16(2):135–45.

[30] Branch DW, Andres R, Digre KB, et al. The association of antiphospholipid antibodies with severe preeclampsia. Obstet Gynecol 1989;73:541–5.

[31] Dekker GA, de Vries JI, Doelitzsch PM, et al. Underlying disorders associated with severe early-onset preeclampsia. Am J Obstet Gynecol 1995;173:1042–8.

[32] Rafla N, Farquharson R. Lupus anticoagulant in preeclampsia and intra-uterine growth retardation. Eur J Obstet Gynecol Reprod Biol 1991;42:167–70.

[33] Miranda-Carus ME, Askanase AD, Clancey RM, et al. Anti-SSA/Ro and anti-SSB/La autoantibodies bind the surface of apoptotic fetal cardiocytes and promote secretion of TNF-alpha by macrophages. J Immunol 2000;165:5345–51.

[34] Provost TT, Watson R, Gammon WR, et al. The neonatal lupus syndrome associated with U1 RNP (nRNP) antibodies. N Engl J Med 1987;315:1135–9.

[35] Goldsmith DP. Neonatal rheumatic disorders. View of the pediatrician. Rheum Dis Clin North Am 1989;15:287–305.

[36] Rider LG, Sherry DD, Glass ST. Neonatal lupus erythematosus simulating transient myasthenia gravis at presentation. J Pediatr 1991;118:417–9.

[37] Dugan EM, Tunnessen WW, Honig PJ, et al. U1RNP antibody-positive neonatal lupus. A report of two cases with immunogenetic studies. Arch Dermatol 1992;128:1490–4.

[38] Sheth AP, Esterly NB, Ratoosh SL, et al. U1RNP positive neonatal lupus erythematosus: association with anti-La antibodies? Br J Dermatol 1995;132:520–6.

[39] Solomon BA, Laude TA, Shalita AR. Neonatal lupus erythematosus: discordant disease expression of U1 RNP-positive antibodies in fraternal twins—is this a subset of neonatal lupus erythematosus or a new distinct syndrome? J Am Acad Dermatol 1995;32:858–62.

[40] Kitridou RC. The neonatal lupus syndrome. In: Wallace DJ, Hahn BH, editors. Dubois' lupus erythematosus. 6th edition. Philadelphia: Lippincott, Williams & Wilkins; 2002. p. 1041–59.

[41] Su CT, Huang CB, Chung MY. Neonatal lupus erythematosus in association with anti-RNP antibody: a case report. Am J Perinatol 2001;18(8):421–6.

[42] Lee LA, Harmon CE, Huff JC, et al. Demonstration of SSA/Ro antigen in human fetal tissues and in neonatal and adult skin. J Invest Dermatol 1985;85:143–6.

[43] Deng JS, Bair LW, Schen-Schwartz S, et al. Localization of Ro (SSA) antigen in the cardiac conduction system. Arthritis Rheum 1987;30:1232–8.

[44] Kitridou RC. The mother in systemic lupus erythematosus. In: Wallace DJ, Hahn BH, editors. Dubois' lupus erythematosus. 6th edition. Philadelphia: Lippincott, Williams & Wilkins; 2002. p. 985–1021.

RHEUMATIC
DISEASE CLINICS
OF NORTH AMERICA

ELSEVIER
SAUNDERS

Rheum Dis Clin N Am 31 (2005) 509–517

Muscle Involvement in Mixed Connective Tissue Disease

Stephen Hall, MBBS, FRACP[a],*,
Patrick Hanrahan, MBBS, FRACP[b]

[a]Department of Medicine, Monash University, Box Hill Hospital, Melbourne, Australia
[b]Goatcher Clinical Research Unit, Royal Perth Hospital, Selby Street,
Shenton Park, WA 6008, Australia

Muscle disease has been recognized as a major feature of mixed connective tissue disease (MCTD) since Sharp's initial description of a distinct clinical-serologic entity with elements of systemic lupus erythematosus (SLE), scleroderma, and polymyositis/dermatomyositis (PM/DM) in 1972 [1]. Even then, the degree and nature of the muscle involvement was ambiguous; 24 out of the 25 patients described having myalgias, but only 72% had "muscle pain, tenderness, weakness and elevated levels of creatine phosphokinase and aldolase." The electromyogram findings were consistent with inflammatory myositis and seven of the eight muscle biopsies that were performed had "inflammatory infiltrates."

Prevalence

The prevalence of myositis in MCTD has varied considerably in different published series. The criteria that were used to diagnose myositis often were not described adequately although it is clear that the presence of myalgia alone is not sufficient to establish a diagnosis. The MCTD classification criteria of Sharp and colleagues [1], Kasukawa and colleagues [2], and Alarcon-Segovia and Cardiel [3] allow a formal diagnosis without muscle involvement. Sharp and colleagues include myositis as one of their five major criteria; however, MCTD can be diagnosed with only four of these or two major criteria plus two minor

---

* Corresponding author. Cabrini Medical Centre, 43/183 Wattletree Road, Malvern, VI 3144, Australia.
  E-mail address: stahall@bigpond.net.au (S. Hall).

criteria as well as antibodies to ribonucleoprotein (RNP)—an obligatory requirement of all criteria) [1]. Alarcon-Segovia and Cardiel [3] require, among other symptoms, either synovitis or myositis from three out of five clinical criteria. Kasukawa and colleagues require one or more clinical features of a constellation of findings in two out of three groups that were described as SLE-like, systemic sclerosis-like, or PM-like. Further, their criteria can be met by just having muscle weakness, elevated levels of creatine kinase, or myogenic pattern on EMG from the PM-like group [2].

In Sharp and colleagues' original series, they concluded that 72% had myositis [1]. In a further report in 1976, Sharp and colleagues [4] stressed the importance of a combination of Raynaud's phenomenon, swollen hands, and myositis in prompting a search for anti-RNP antibodies; 63% of 100 patients who had antibodies to RNP had myositis. Alarcon-Segovia [5] assessed 100 patients who had MCTD and found myositis in 55%. This was similar to the presence of myositis in 53% of 30 patients who were studied by Kitridou and colleagues [6]. Myositis was not defined, but was confirmed pathologically in 6 of the 16 patients. Amigues and colleagues [7] applied the different criteria to 45 patients who were selected on the basis of a positive anti-RNP; only 15.6% had myositis. Burdt and colleagues' [8] data from 47 patients who met Kasukawa and colleagues' criteria were more consistent with most of the other series; 51% had myositis. It is reasonable to conclude that the prevalence of myositis in MCTD is between 50% and 70%.

Clinical description

Myositis tends to be a feature of MCTD in the earlier phases of the disease; it is the presenting symptom only rarely. The largest long-term study of MCTD reviewed the progress of 47 patients who had well-documented disease with at least 3 consecutive years of follow-up (mean follow-up 15 years). Only 2% manifested myositis at presentation. Eventually, 51% developed myositis, although at final evaluation only 6% still had active myositis [8]. It has been suggested that myositis of MCTD may be milder and more responsive to treatment than PM/DM [9,10].

Detailed clinical descriptions of myositis in MCTD are sparse; it generally is believed that MCTD-related myositis is similar in its clinical presentation to other inflammatory myopathies. Thus, patients present with generalized weakness, but little, if any, wasting. The pelvic girdle musculature is affected more than the shoulder girdles, and the usual symptomatic complaints include difficulty arising from a low chair, climbing stairs, and working with the arms held above the head. The extraocular muscles are spared although neck extensors can be involved and weakness of extension may produce a "dropped head syndrome."

Severity is variable and ranges from mild to disabling. Focal forms of myositis in MCTD have been described; one case presented as a mass in the neck that simulated jugular thrombophlebitis [11].

Respiratory symptoms that are due to diaphragmatic dysfunction have been reported in MCTD myositis [12]. Dysphagia may occur in MCTD-related myositis because of involvement of the esophageal striated muscle [13]; myocarditis has been reported in several patients who had MCTD myositis [14].

Dalakas and Hohlfeld [15] proposed that only DM can be associated with MCTD (in the sense that classification criteria for both are met) and "overlap" with MCTD by sharing some characteristics of both diseases, whereas PM can overlap with a wide spectrum of other connective tissue diseases, but not scleroderma or MCTD.

Myalgia is common in MCTD [1,7], even in the absence of myositis. Sharp and colleagues' original series suggests that it may be more common than in PM and DM; however, myalgia alone is an insufficient basis for proposing the presence of myositis and may be explained by other conditions (eg, fibromyalgia) that could coexist with MCTD and may be overrepresented in this population, as has been seen in SLE [16]. The finding of diffuse muscular pain and a mildly increased creatine kinase level should not be assumed to indicate the presence of myositis. Further laboratory confirmation, including a positive muscle biopsy, should be sought before committing patients to immunosuppressive therapies.

In addition, a variety of other conditions can be confused with myositis on clinical, laboratory, or pathologic grounds. These include muscular dystrophies (eg, recently-described dysferlin gene mutations), metabolic myopathies that can appear inflammatory on biopsy specimens obtained after episodes of rhabdomyolysis, acid maltase deficiency, and endocrine myopathies. Recently, these were reviewed in detail [17].

Pathology

Currently-used pathologic techniques usually allow a clear distinction of DM from PM, although the latter can be confused with inclusion body myositis [15]. In DM, there is an inflammatory infiltrate of $CD4^+$ cells around blood vessels and in the septae; membrane attack complex in capillaries often is detectable before any inflammatory changes in muscle are evident. As a consequence, there is capillary loss, microinfarcts, and perifascicular atrophy [18]. In PM, the inflammatory infiltrate invades the muscle fibers with a predominance of $CD8^+$ T cells surrounding and invading muscle cells that overexpress major histocompatibility complex (MHC)-I antigen; the resultant $CD8^+$/MHC-I complex is believed to be characteristic of PM [19].

In Sharp and colleagues' early report [1], 7 out of 8 patients had "inflammatory infiltrates present" on muscle biopsy. One of these that was reported in more detail "showed focal interstitial myositis" that was consistent with the known histology of PM at the time. In 1977, Oxenhandler and colleagues, including Sharp, described muscle biopsies from 13 patients who had

MCTD [20]. Eight showed a lymphocytic infiltrate; in 4 patients this was described as a "lymphocytic vasculitis." This also was before a pathologic distinction between PM and DM was recognized [21]; no attempt was made to dichotomize the findings which resulted in difficulty in interpreting their report. Perifascicular atrophy was seen in 3 patients, and 7 patients had focal fiber necrosis (ie, features of DM and PM were seen, possibly in different biopsies although this is not clear). Cooke and Lurie [22] reported one case with a biopsy that showed perivascular and interstitial infiltration of inflammatory cells. They noted that "these changes are believed to be compatible with polymyositis"; however, the patient had the violaceous rash of DM and their comment reflects the concept, at the time, that DM was essentially PM with a rash, with no need to differentiate the pathology. Bennett and O'Connell [23] reported, in detail, 20 patients who had MCTD; only 4 patients had a muscle biopsy, although 7 (35%) patients were believed to have had myositis. All showed perivascular inflammatory infiltration and one biopsy had "fibre degeneration with infiltrations of neutrophils and plasma cells." None of the biopsied patients was reported to have the skin changes of DM. The difficulty of reporting muscle biopsies accurately—combined with the lack of understanding of the significance of perivascular inflammation and the need to differentiate perimysial from endomysial infiltration—renders these earlier descriptions less helpful in understanding the nature of the inflammation in the myositis of MCTD than otherwise would have been the case.

Lundberg and colleagues [10] compared biopsies from a group of 29 patients who had PM, DM, or myositis that was associated with another connective tissue disease (CTD). Seven of the 13 patients in the last group were anti-RNP positive and met criteria for MCTD. Twenty-eight patients had at least one muscle biopsy. Patients who had PM had lymphocytic infiltration—predominantly in the endomysium around the muscle fibers—and, in some cases, invading the fibers (typical of PM). In DM and MCTD (as well as the anti-RNP negative group that had "other CTD"), the lymphocytes had a perimysial distribution (ie, the biopsies most resembled DM).

Vianna and colleagues [24] used current immunohistologic techniques to suggest that the pathology of the myositis in MCTD is unique and shares features of DM and PM. Fourteen patients who had MCTD were compared with 8 who had PM, 5 who had DM, and 4 who had other diseases. MCTD biopsies showed a heterogeneous distribution with perivascular and endomysial infiltration with lymphocytes. Although vascular density of MCTD biopsies was reduced to levels that were comparable to DM—in contrast to subjects who had PM and in whom vascular density was normal—little detectable membrane attack complex was seen in vessel walls and only low levels of adhesion molecules were seen in the vessels; these findings would have been expected in DM. Their conclusion is that, like DM, MCTD probably is a humorally mediated disease with a major involvement of blood vessels, although there are sufficient components of DM and PM to suggest that there may be a characteristic muscle pathology in MCTD. This hypothesis would benefit from confirmation in further series.

On balance, pathologic studies have not allowed a definite conclusion; however, the pathology in MCTD most likely is related more closely to that of DM than PM.

Other forms of myopathy have been described in overlap syndromes, including a necrotizing myopathy with pipestem capillaries that was described by Emslie-Smith and Engel [25]; a patient may develop features of an inflammatory myopathy with minimal inflammatory infiltrate, deposition of membrane attack complex in vessels, and a characteristic "pipestem" appearance of vessels. Such changes have been seen in one patient who had typical MCTD [26] and in another patient who had a scleroderma-type overlap CTD [27]. This pattern is recognized increasingly; one study suggested that 19% of patients who formerly were considered to have PM have this entity which may occur in the context of malignancy or CTD [28].

Myositis and antibodies

Autoantibodies to RNP (anti-U1-snRNP) are an obligatory feature of MCTD, and therefore, are found in all patients who have MCTD with myositis. They are not specific to MCTD and also may occur in isolated inflammatory muscle disease. Brouwer and colleagues [29] found these U1 RNP antibodies in the sera of 25 of 417 (6%) patients who had myositis from 11 European countries. Seventeen of 198 patients (8.6%) who had PM, 7 of 181 patients (3.9%) who had DM, and 1 of 38 patients (2.6%) who had inclusion body myositis had detectable antibody. In a Canadian series, 10% of patients who had inflammatory myopathy possessed antibody to U1 RNP [30].

Treatment

Because inflammatory myopathies are rare diseases, they have been subject to few clinical trials. The myositis of MCTD has never been addressed specifically in a clinical trial; treatment generally follows the guidelines for treatment of PM/DM.

Corticosteroids are the initial treatment of choice. Typically, this is instituted in high doses, using the equivalent of 60 to 100 mg/day of prednisone, although this may present specific problems in the context of MCTD. In at least one case, such therapy precipitated a scleroderma-type renal crisis with malignant hypertension and rapidly progressive renal failure [26]. This underscores the need for scrupulous attention to blood pressure control with high-dose corticosteroid therapy in MCTD.

Second-line therapies for patients who have inflammatory myopathies and respond poorly to corticosteroid therapy include high-dose intravenous gamma globulin; a variety of immunosuppressant agents, including azathioprine, methotrexate, alkylators, cyclosporin, tacrolimus, mycophelylate mofetil, and tumor necrosis factor inhibitors; and experimental therapies, such as stem cell transplantation (reviewed recently in [31]). Few of these have been studied systematically in the idiopathic inflammatory myopathies of PM and DM; none has been addressed specifically in the myositis of MCTD.

High-dose immunoglobulin therapy was effective in improving power, functional state, and muscle histology in clinical trials in patients who had DM [32]. The presence of immunoglobulin deposits on biopsy with vascular changes that are akin to DM suggests a specific rationale for the use of immunoglobulin therapy in the myositis of MCTD.

Autologous peripheral blood stem cell transplantation has been used in a variety of treatment-resistant immunologic diseases, including the myositis of MCTD. A 65-year-old man who had MCTD and significant myositis that was resistant to high-dose corticosteroids, azathioprine, and intravenous pulse corticosteroids coupled with cyclophosphamide, received such a transplant. At 21 months, there was improvement in his ability to self-care although there was only slight improvement in muscle strength. Creatine kinase levels essentially were unchanged after the procedure, and electromyography and muscle biopsies continued to show active myositis with necrosis; this suggested that there had been a modest response, at best, to such aggressive therapy [33].

Prognosis

The myositis of MCTD may be milder and generally more responsive to treatment than idiopathic inflammatory myopathies. One study from France suggested that possession of the characteristic autoantibody of MCTD, anti-U1 RNP, indicated a more benign prognosis. Five of 91 patients who had myositis had anti-U1 RNP antibodies. All five manifested typical features of myopathy with weakness, increased creatine kinase levels, and abnormal muscle biopsy. All responded well to corticosteroid therapy, although two relapsed and also required the use of methotrexate. This was a more satisfactory response rate than was seen in the remaining patients of this series [9].

Lundberg and colleagues [10] found that patients who had myositis and antibody to RNP—although having similar degrees of muscle weakness, erythrocyte sedimentation rate, and creatine kinase levels—had lesser histopathologic changes on muscle biopsy. Six of seven patients who had anti-RNP antibodies were able to have corticosteroid therapy withdrawn because their myositis was in complete remission. These findings are in keeping with the long-term observational studies of MCTD which found that only 6% of patients who had MCTD had active myositis at a mean of 15 years of follow-up [8].

Several series have addressed the relationship between malignancy and myositis. The Bohan and Peter [34,35] classification of myositis, which differentiates between myositis of malignancy and myositis associated with CTD, implies a lack of association with malignancy in cases of myositis that occur in the context of a CTD, which would include MCTD.

A population-based series of 537 cases of biopsy-proven inflammatory myopathy with diagnosis based on histopathologic criteria suggested that although DM was associated more closely with risk of malignancy (standardized incidence ratio of 6.2; CI, 3.9–10.0), an increased risk also was seen in patients who had CTD (standardized incidence ratio of 4.6; CI, 1.2–11.7) [36]. Patients were not characterized according to the type of CTD. The generalizability of this observation remains to be confirmed as does a more precise classification of the nature of the CTDs that may be "at risk." At this stage, there seems little justification for intensive cancer screening.

Summary

Myositis is common in MCTD. The pathology of such involvement tends to be more similar to that seen in DM than in PM though some overlap is apparent. In the absence of clinical trials specifically directed at the myositis of MCTD, patients should be treated in the manner recommended for other forms of myositis. Myositis of MCTD may enjoy a better prognosis than other forms of myositis.

References

[1] Sharp GC, Irvin WS, Tan EM, et al. Mixed connective tissue disease: an apparently distinct rheumatic disease syndrome associated with a specific antibody to an extractible nuclear antigen (ENA). Am J Med 1972;52:148–59.
[2] Kasukawa R, Tojo T, Miyawaki S. Preliminary diagnostic criteria for classification of mixed connective tissue disease. In: Kasukawa R, Sharp GC, editors. Mixed connective tissue disease and anti-nuclear antibodies. Amsterdam: Elsevier; 1987. p. 41–7.
[3] Alarcon-Segovia D, Cardiel MH. Comparison between three diagnostic criteria for mixed connective tissue disease. Study of 593 patients. J Rheum 1989;16:328–34.
[4] Sharp GC, Irvin WS, May CM, et al. Association of antibodies to ribonucleoprotein and Sm antigens with mixed connective tissue disease, systemic lupus erythematosus and other rheumatic diseases. N Engl J Med 1976;295:1150–4.
[5] Alarcon-Segovia D. Mixed connective tissue disease and overlap syndromes. Clin Dermatol 1994;12:309–16.
[6] Kitridou RC, Akmal M, Turkel SB, et al. Renal involvement in mixed connective tissue disease: a longitudinal clinicopathologic study. Semin Arthritis Rheum 1986;16:135–45.
[7] Amigues JM, Cantagrel A, Abbal M, et al. Comparative study of 4 diagnosis criteria sets for mixed connective tissue disease in patients with anti-RNP antibodies. J Rheumatol 1996;23: 2055–62.
[8] Burdt MA, Hoffman RW, Deutscher SL, et al. Long-term outcome in mixed connective tissue disease: longitudinal clinical and serologic findings. Arthritis Rheum 1999;42:899–909.
[9] Coppo P, Clauvel JP, Bengoufa D, et al. Inflammatory myositis associated with anti-U1-small nuclear ribonucleoprotein antibodies: a subset of myositis associated with a favourable outcome. Rheumatol 2002;41:1040–6.
[10] Lundberg I, Nennesmo I, Hedfors E. A clinical, serological and histopathological study of

myositis patients with and without anti-RNP antibodies. Semin Arthritis Rheum 1992;22: 127–38.

[11] Rivest C, Miller FW, Love LA, et al. Focal myositis presenting as pseudothrombophlebitis of the neck in a patient with mixed connective tissue disease. Arthritis Rheum 1996;39: 1254–8.

[12] Martens J, Demedts M. Diaphragmatic dysfunction in mixed connective tissue disease. Scand J Rheumatol 1982;11:165–7.

[13] Alpert MA, Goldberg SH, Singsen BH, et al. Cardiovascular manifestations of mixed connective tissue disease in adults. Circulation 1983;68:1182–93.

[14] Lash AD, Wittman A-L, Quismorio FP. Myocarditis in mixed connective tissue disease: clinical and pathological study of three cases and review of the literature. Semin Arthritis Rheum 1986; 15:288–96.

[15] Dalakas MC, Hohlfeld R. Polymyositis and dermatomyositis. Lancet 2003;362:971–82.

[16] Friedman AW, Tewi MB, Ahan C, et al. Systemic lupus erythematosus in three ethnic groups; XV. Prevalence and correlates of fibro myalgia. Lupus 2003;12:274–9.

[17] Nirmalanathan M, Holton JL, Hanna MG. Is it really myositis? A consideration of the differential diagnosis. Curr Opin Rheumatol 2004;16:684–91.

[18] Kissel JT, Mendell JR, Rammohan KW. Microvascular deposition of complement membrane attack complex in dermatomyositis. N Engl J Med 1986;314:329–34.

[19] Arahata K, Engel AG. Monoclonal antibody analysis of mononuclear cells in myopathies: V, identification and quantitation of T8+ cytotoxic and T8 suppressor cells. Ann Neurol 1988; 23:493–9.

[20] Oxenhandler R, Hart M, Corman L, et al. Pathology of skeletal muscle in mixed connective tissue disease. Arthritis Rheum 1977;20:985–8.

[21] Bronner IM, Linssen WHJP, Van der Meulen MFG, et al. Polymyositis. Arch Neurol 2004;61: 132–5.

[22] Cooke CL, Lurie HI. Case report: fatal gastrointestinal haemorrhage in mixed connective tissue disease. Arthritis Rheum 1977;20:1421–7.

[23] Bennett RM, O'Connell DJ. Mixed connective tissue disease: a clinicopathological study. Semin Arthritis Rheum 1980;10:25–51.

[24] Vianna MAAG, Borges CTL, Borba EF, et al. Myositis in mixed connective tissue disease: a unique syndrome characterized by immunohistopathologic elements of both polymyositis and dermatomyositis. Arq Neuropsiquiatr 2004;62:923–34.

[25] Emslie-Smith AM, Engel AG. Necrotizing myopathy with pipestem capillaries, microvascular deposition of the complement membrane attack complex (MAC) and minimal cellular infiltration. Neurology 1991;41:936–9.

[26] Greenberg SA, Amato AA. Inflammatory myopathy associated with mixed connective tissue disease and scleroderma renal crisis. Muscle Nerve 2001;24:1562–6.

[27] De Bleecker J, Ver Vaet V, Van den Berg HP. Necrotizing myopathy with microvascular deposition of the complement membrane attack complex. Clin Neuropathol 2004;23:76–9.

[28] Van der Meulen MF, Bronner IM, Hoogendijk JE, et al. Polymyositis: a diagnostic entity reconsidered. Neurology 2003;61:316–21.

[29] Brouwer R, Hengtsman GJD, Vree Egberts W, et al. Autoantibody profile in the sera of European patients with myositis. Ann Rheum Dis 2001;60:116–23.

[30] Uthman I, Vazquez-Abad D, Senecal J-L. Distinctive features of idiopathic inflammatory myopathies in French Canadians. Semin Arthritis Rheum 1996;26:447–58.

[31] Amato AA, Griggs RC. Treatment of idiopathic inflammatory myopathies. Curr Opin Neurol 2003;16:569–75.

[32] Dalakas MC, Illa I, Dambrosia JM, et al. A controlled clinical trial of high-dose intravenous immune globulin infusions as treatment for dermatomyositis. N Engl J Med 1993;329: 1993–2000.

[33] Myllykangas-Luosujarvi R, Jantunen E, Kaipiainen-Seppanen O, et al. Autologous peripheral blood stem cell transplantation in a patient with severe mixed connective tissue disease. Scand J Rheumatol 2000;29:326–7.

[34] Bohan A, Peter JB. Polymyositis and dermatomyositis (first of two parts). N Engl J Med 1975;
     292:344–7.
[35] Bohan A, Peter JB. Polymyositis and dermatomyositis (second of two parts). N Engl J Med
     1975;292:403–7.
[36] Buchbinder R, Forbes A, Hall S, et al. Incidence of malignant disease in biopsy-proven
     inflammatory myopathy. Ann Intern Med 2001;134:1087–95.

ELSEVIER
SAUNDERS

Rheum Dis Clin N Am 31 (2005) 519–533

RHEUMATIC
DISEASE CLINICS
OF NORTH AMERICA

Other Manifestations of Mixed Connective Tissue Disease

Janet E. Pope, MD, MPH, FRCPC*

*Divisions of Rheumatology and Epidemiology and Biostatistics, Department of Medicine,
Faculty of Medicine, University of Western Ontario, 1151 Richmond Street, London,
ON N6A 5B8, Canada*

This article describes other manifestations of mixed connective tissue disease (MCTD), focusing on inflammatory arthritis, the gastrointestinal (GI) tract (the esophagus in particular), the kidney, skin, and hematologic changes such as thrombocytopenia. Inflammatory arthritis is common in MCTD, often mimicking rheumatoid arthritis, and in many cases erosions are seen on radiographs. Human leukocyte antigen (HLA)-DR4 is associated with polyarthritis in MCTD. Esophageal dysmotility is common in MCTD and similar to, but often not as severe as, that found in scleroderma. Renal involvement is less common and can include nephrotic syndrome, glomerulonephritis, and, rarely, renal crisis. Pericarditis has been associated with MCTD but often is occult and not diagnosed until postmortem. Conduction abnormalities and autonomic neuropathy can occur, affecting the heart. Skin involvement can mimic systemic lupus erythematosus (SLE), including discoidlike lesions and subacute cutaneous lupus. Although the biopsies in patients who have MCTD are similar to subacute cutaneous or discoid lupus, vasculopathy and more bland infiltrates are seen with MCTD. Thrombocytopenia can be severe, particularly when it is immune mediated and when it occurs with thrombocytopenia purpura (TTP). Other rare autoimmune conditions, such as myasthenia gravis, can be associated with MCTD. Due to the complexity of potential organ involvements in MCTD, vigilance with appropriate diagnosis and treatment is warranted.

* Division of Rheumatology, St. Joseph's Health Care London, 258 Grosvenor Street, London, ON N6A 4V2, Canada.
E-mail address: janet.pope@sjhc.london.on.ca

0889-857X/05/$ – see front matter © 2005 Elsevier Inc. All rights reserved.
doi:10.1016/j.rdc.2005.04.011   *rheumatic.theclinics.com*

Joint involvement in mixed connective tissue disease

Arthritis is a common feature with MCTD. It is often polyarticular, can be rheumatoid arthritis (RA)-like, and can have features of erosive arthritis on radiographs. Rheumatoid nodules can occur; and less frequently, calcinosis and digital tuft or pulp resorption occur. There have been reports of crystal-associated arthritis in patients who have MCTD (hydroxyapatite and gout), accompanying seronegative arthritis, and what looked like juvenile arthritis that was poly-articular in two children and evolved into MCTD. Anti–U1-RNP antibody may be a predictor of more aggressive erosive arthritis. Avascular necrosis (AVN) has also been reported to occur in MCTD. It is difficult to know the true prevalence of inflammatory and erosive arthritis in MCTD because there are no population studies. Prospective studies and case series may over-report due to case ascer-tainment biases (referral bias).

Inflammatory arthritis is often a presenting feature in MCTD. Bennet [1] described 20 patients who had MCTD, of whom 11 presented with inflammatory arthritis. Six of the 11 patients who had arthritis had deformities, and erosions were characteristic, often small, and occasionally asymmetrical. Another case series demonstrated that 27 of 28 people who had MCTD had joint involvement [2]. The author described 25 of 28 patients who were rheumatoid factor positive, five patients who had rheumatoid nodules, and 26 of 27 patients who had radiographs with abnormal findings. Twelve patients had erosive arthritis, and six patients had calcinosis. Therefore, many had RA-like features with symmetrical polyarticular synovitis, whereas others had systemic sclerosis-like changes. Another article [3] described 17 of 19 patients with MCTD having inflammatory arthritis, of whom eight patients were initially misdiagnosed with rheumatoid arthritis. Thirty-five percent had RA-like hand deformities and contractures, and decreased range of motion occurred in 47%. Thirty percent had erosions or cystic change on x-rays. Radiographs of 20 patients who had MCTD revealed 12 pa-tients with erosive arthritis [4]. Another radiologic series in MCTD ($n = 10$) demonstrated 80% with periarticular osteopenia, 70% with erosive arthritis, and 60% with digital tuft resorption. A further 20% had subluxations. Thus, the ra-diographs had features of rheumatoid arthritis and sclerodermalike changes [5].

Non-erosive Jaccoud's arthropathy has been described in MCTD in a case report [6]. This patients disease looked more like lupus arthropathy on x-ray than RA.

Catoggio and colleagues [7] compared 34 patients who had scleroderma with nine patients who had MCTD. Calcinosis, distal pulp atrophy, and digital tuft resorption were more common in scleroderma (50%). However, in the patients who had MCTD, there was more erosive arthritis. The patients who had MCTD were younger at age of onset but had similar disease duration to scleroderma, and erosions were positively correlated with the presence of a rheumatoid factor. Findings were similar in scleroderma and MCTD, but the prevalences were different between groups with respect to digital resorption and erosive arthritis.

Table 1
Studies of frequency of erosive arthritis in mixed connective tissue disease

First author, year [Ref.]	Total no. of patients	No. of patients who had arthritis (%)	No. of patients who had arthritis with erosions (%)
Bennett, 1978 [1]	20	11 (55)	6/11 (55)
Ramos-Niembro, 1979 [2]	28	27 (96)	12/27 (44)
Halla, 1978 [3]	10	10 (100)	7/10 (70)
O'Connell, 1977 [4]	19	17 (89)	5/17 (30)
Udoff, 1977 [5]	20	20 (100)	12/20 (60)

Other features of arthritis and the occurrence of rheumatoid nodules have been described in MCTD [7]. There are also cases of arthritis mutilans, which occurs more commonly in psoriatic arthritis [1,8]. A 55-year-old woman with 8 years of MCTD with Raynaud's, arthritis, digital ulcers with gangrene, restrictive lung disease, and esophagitis developed atlantoaxial subluxation. She was anti–U1-RNP positive. One would expect this type of subluxation to occur in RA or ankylosing spondylitis and less likely SLE, but it can occur in MCTD [9].

There are descriptions of gout in MCTD and hydroxyapatite crystal deposition [10,11]. There is also a case report in the literature describing a man with long-standing ankylosing spondylitis who later developed Sjögren's symptoms and swollen hands with myositis. He was positive for anti-Ro and anti–U1-RNP antibodies [12]. Due to a paucity of reports such as this, it may have been coincidental in a patient who was HLA-B27 positive and who was anti–U1-RNP positive; the latter increasing the risk of MCTD. Another patient has been described who was 26 years of age and who had mandibular retrognathism from condylosis with features of polyarthritis, morning stiffness, subcutaneous nodules, acrosclerosis, and parotid swelling [13]. She was negative for rheumatoid factor and positive for ANA and anti-double stranded DNA and was diagnosed with MCTD. Thus, retrognathism may accompany MCTD.

Two children (one was 3 years of age, and the other was 15 years of age) with presumed juvenile rheumatoid arthritis developed MCTD with destructive arthritis [14]. AVN has also been rarely reported in MCTD [1].

In a series of 540 patients who were positive for ANA, 21 had anti–U1-RNP antibodies. These patients had polyarthritis with more aggressive erosive arthritis [15]. Arthritis in MCTD is most common at the wrists (followed by the meta-carpophalangeal joint, the proximal interphalangeal [PIP] joint, and the metatarsophalangeal joint), and up to 70% had x-ray erosions (in the 21 patients who were positive for anti-U1-RNP). Table 1 demonstrates the frequency of erosive arthritis in MCTD from some of the published case series.

Gastrointestinal involvement in mixed connective tissue disease

Most areas of the GI tract can be involved in MCTD, particularly esophageal dysmotility. Autoimmune hepatitis, primary biliary cirrhosis, pancreatitis vasculitis, and GI vasculitis have been reported. There are case reports of pneumatosis intestinalis and protein losing enteropathy in MCTD. The seroprevalence of *Helicobacter pylori* may be higher in MCTD compared with a healthy population.

Some authors have thought that the GI involvement in MCTD is virtually indistinguishable from scleroderma [16,17]. Several case series describe the esophageal manifestations in MCTD [18–23]. Gastroesophageal reflux, dyspepsia, dysphagia, and abnormal esophageal manometry are common.

Marshall [18] reported observations of 61 patients with MCTD. Forty-eight percent had heartburn, and 38% dysphagia. Forty-three percent had upper esophageal manometry abnormalities, whereas 26% had no esophageal abnormalities. He also noted constipation in three patients, diarrhea in five patients, and vomiting in two patients. There were rare occurrences of conditions such as chronic active hepatitis, pancreatitis, malabsorption, and vasculitis (one of each) in this series [18]. Another cohort of 21 people who had MCTD was described where esophageal dysphagia occurred in 19%, dyspepsia occurred in 24%, and abnormal esophageal motility occurred in 85% [19]. They observed that the lower esophageal sphincter (LES) pressure in MCTD was significantly lower than in healthy control subjects but that the mean LES pressure was higher (ie, less impaired) than in scleroderma. Pharyngeal dysphagia was a complaint in 24% of this population. They concluded that although esophageal involvement in MCTD was similar in frequency, it was slightly different from that seen in scleroderma. Seventeen patients who had MCTD were compared with 14 patients who had SLE [20]. Dyspepsia and gastroesophageal reflux disease were found in 11 of 17 patients who had MCTD, and 10 of 11 patients had significant abnormal manometry. Severe peristaltic abnormalities were found in nine patients who had MCTD. They hypothesized that Raynaud's phenomenon and esophageal abnormal peristalsis were correlated and that esophageal dysmotility was more pronounced in MCTD than in SLE. Lapadula and colleagues [21] studied esophageal motility disorders in 150 patients who had rheumatic diseases, of whom 17 patients had MCTD. Contrary to the article by Guttierez and colleagues [20], Lapadula and colleagues [21] reported that Raynaud's was likely pathogenetically not related to esophageal motility disorders. Eighty-eight percent of the patients who had MCTD had abnormal esophageal manometry [21]. In a smaller series, 12 patients who had MCTD were studied, of whom three patients had an abnormal barium swallow radiographs, half had abnormal esophageal manometry, and 6 of 12 patients complained of dysphagia [22]. Stacher [23] published data on six patients who had MCTD. All six patients had abnormal lower esophageal sphincter pressures with esophageal dysfunction, and five had other autonomic dysfunction especially cardiac changes.

Five children and adolescents who had MCTD have been characterized [24]. Most of these patients had reflux, and abnormal intraesophageal pH monitoring was found in these patients. Weston [25] studied GI motility in MCTD ($n = 8$) and found many abnormalities similar to those reported in scleroderma.

Other gastrointestinal manifestations

Rarely, autoimmune hepatitis is associated with MCTD [26,27]. An autopsy series of livers in patients who died of autoimmune diseases, including 11 patients who had MCTD, revealed one patient who had autoimmune hepatitis and one patient who had primary biliary cirrhosis [26]. None of the MCTD specimens had arteritis, although arteritis was found in some specimens from patients who had died from polyarteritis nodosa. There is a case report of duodenal hemorrhage from vasculitis in a patient who had MCTD with skin involvement including leukocytoclastic vasculitis [28]. This is likely rare in MCTD.

Scleroderma is at times associated with pneumatosis intestinalis with pseudo-diverticulum. There have been at least four cases reported of this occurring in the large bowel in MCTD [29,30]. Pancreatitis from MCTD seems to be rare [27].

There has been a case report of protein-losing gastroenteropathy associated with MCTD [31]. This was successfully treated with cyclophosphamide. Bowel vasculitis, protein-losing gastroenteropathy, and (rarely) esophageal dysmotility may be responsive to steroids or immunosuppressives [18,28,31].

H pylori infection can cause dyspepsia and ulcers. A study compared *H pylori* IgG antibodies in RA, SLE, polymyositis, scleroderma, MCTD, and Sjögren's syndrome with healthy volunteers and with patients who had chronic obstructive pulmonary disease [32]. *H pylori* antibody levels were high in cases of Sjögren's syndrome and were slightly elevated in MCTD compared with healthy control subjects. It is uncertain whether gastritis and *H pylori* infection (past or current) was present.

In summary, GI symptoms and signs are common in MCTD, particularly in those related to esophageal dysmotility and abnormal lower esophageal sphincter tone. Table 2 illustrates some of the larger series of upper GI manifestations in MCTD.

Sjögren's syndrome in mixed connective tissue disease

When MCTD was initially described by Sharp [33], the frequency of accompanying Sjögren's syndrome was low. Over time it has been appreciated

Table 2
Upper gastrointestinal manifestation studies in mixed connective tissue disease

| First author, year [Ref.] | Total no. of patients | Patients who had | | |
		Dyspepsia	Dysphagia	Abnormal esophageal manometry
Marshall, 1990 [18]	61	48%	38%	43%
Doria, 1991 [19]	21	24%	19%	85%
Gutierrez, 1982 [20]	17	65%	53%	59%[a]
Lapadula, 1994 [21]	17	—	—	88%
Dantas, 1985 [22]	12	—	50%	50%

[a] 10 of 11 studied were abnormal.

that Sjögren's syndrome, including sicca symptoms of dry eyes, dry mouth, and salivary and lacrimal gland inflammation, is relatively common [34–37]. Fifty-five patients who had MCTD have been described, of whom 43% had sicca complaints, 33% were anti-Ro antibody positive, and 4% had anti-La antibody [34]. Anti-Ro antibody correlated positively with photosensitivity ($P < .001$). Ninety-four percent of patients who had MCTD ($n = 19$) compared with 80% of subjects who had RA and 58% of subjects who had ankylosing spondylitis were found to have Sjögren's syndrome with focal sialadenitis, abnormal Schirmer's tests, or changes on minor salivary gland biopsy [35]. In Mexico, Alarcon-Segovia [36] described 12 of 25 patients who had MCTD who had xerostomia or ocular dryness with keratoconjunctivitis sicca. Erosive TMJ arthritis has also been found in patients with Sjögren's-associated symptoms in MCTD [37]. Nine of 10 patients described in that series had complaints of Sjögren's symptoms. Table 3 demonstrates the frequency of Sjögren's symptomatology in MCTD, which ranges from 42% to 94%.

Other rare symptoms, such as trigeminal neuralgia, neuropathy, and lymphadenopathy, have been reported in a patient who had MCTD and Sjögren's syndrome [38]. There have also been case reports of Sjögren's syndrome concomitant with MCTD and autoimmune hepatitis [39,40].

In Sjögren's syndrome, there is an increased risk of lymphoma, but pseudolymphoma can occur with lymphocytic collections that could be mistaken for a malignant tumor. There is a case report of a woman who had MCTD who had an abdominal pseudolymphoma and sicca complaints [41]. We can conclude that Sjögren's symptoms can be common in MCTD. Most series have not studied the frequency of anti-Ro and anti-La antibodies in patients with Sjögren's syndrome compared with those without in MCTD.

Hameenkorpi and colleagues [42] noted that there is more hypergammaglobulinemia in MCTD than in scleroderma. Hypergammaglobulinemia is also common in Sjögren's syndrome. These authors also observed an increase of HLA-DR4 and MCTD compared with some other connective tissue diseases. This could be why there is an erosive inflammatory symmetrical polyarthritis commonly found in MCTD because HLA-DR4 is commonly associated with RA and yields a bad prognosis.

Table 3
Studies of frequency of Sjogren's in mixed connective tissue disease

First author, year [Ref.]	Total no. of patients	Anti-Ro–positive	Anti-La–positive	Sicca symptoms
Setty, 2002 [34]	55	33%	4%	42%
Helenius, 2001 [35]	19	—	—	94%
Alarcon, 1976 [36]	25	—	—	48%
Konttinen, 1990 [37]	10	—	—	90%

Cutaneous manifestations of mixed connective tissue disease

Patients who have MCTD can have photosensitivity, inflammatory rash, livedo reticularis, and calcinosis. Anti-Ro antibody is correlated with some lupus-like cutaneous manifestations [34]. Many people who have MCTD have puffy hands. Fig. 1 illustrates a patient who has MCTD whose hands have improved over time. He has periungual dilated capillaries around the nail beds and one area of infarct. He also has inflammatory arthritis, polymyositis, anticardiolipin antibody with pulmonary embolism, and a low white blood cell count.

It has been postulated that livedoid vasculitis in MCTD is associated with a poor prognosis [43]. A description of a 21-year-old woman with 2 years of MCTD has been published [43]. This patient rapidly developed ulcers consistent with livedoid vasculitis accompanied by Raynaud's phenomenon and polyarthritis and swollen hands. She had a strongly positive ANA and anti-RNP and was HLA-DR4 and DR53 positive. She developed disseminated intervascular coagulation and died. Fig. 2 illustrates the hands of a patient with cutaneous vasculitis on the palms and, in particular, the distal fingers.

Cutaneous eruptions in eight patients with connective tissue disease were biopsied [44]. The lesions were in light-exposed areas and were erythematosus, annular, or papulosquamous. Five of eight patients mimicked subacute cutaneous lupus. One patient had several telangiectasias and a scaly patch on the face, another had palpable purpura, and a third had dorsal hand blisters similar to porphyria cutaneous tarda. Most biopsies revealed a cell-poor or lichenoid inter-faced dermatitis with necrotic keratinocytes. There was an absence of peri-vascular extravasation and follicular plugging. Thus, the biopsies were similar to subacute cutaneous lupus. They could be distinguished from subacute cutaneous lupus because they had vascular ectasia, hypovascularity, or luminal thrombosis. The biopsy of one patient was compatible with pustular leukocyto-clastic vasculitis. Two of eight biopsies had positive lupus band tests [44]. In vivo speckled nuclear staining from immunoglobulin (nuclear staining of kera-

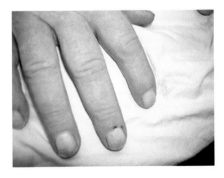

Fig. 1. The hand of a man who has MCTD. Note the puffy fingers and slight erythema of the skin. There is also periungual nail change on the 3rd finger and fusiform PIP swelling from inflammatory arthritis.

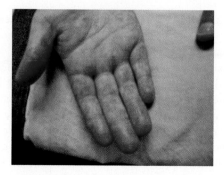

Fig. 2. The hand of a woman who has livedoid vasculitis. There is a livedo reticularislike pattern with distal fingertip palmar erythema. Note the plaquelike changes at the mid-phalanx of the 2nd and 3rd fingers and the 3rd finger proximally.

tinocytes for IgG and complement) correlated with antibodies to RNP and Ro. The microangiopathy of the MCTD cutaneous lesions is distinct from subacute cutaneous lupus. The leukocytoclastic vasculitis and MCTD has been ascribed to an Arthus type III reaction to circulating immune complexes.

Two patients were found to have discoid lupus for several years before the development of MCTD [45]. Each had high anti-RNP antibody titers and nuclear staining by direct immunofluorescence of normal skin. Bentley-Phillips [46] published a case series of four African women with MCTD manifest as

Table 4
Involvement of other organ systems in mixed connective tissue disease

Organ system	Manifestations
Cutaneous	Livedo reticularis[a]
	Livedoid vasculitis
	Subacute cutaneous lupuslike skin changes
	Telangectasia[a]
	Pustular leucocytoclastic vasculitis
	Discoid lupus
Hematologic	Anticardiolipin antibodies 15%–18%
	(not usually β2-glycoprotein-1)
	Thrombotic thrombocytic purpura
	Thrombocytopenia
	Hemolytic anemia
Renal involvement	Membranous glomerular nephritis[b]
	Mesangial glomerular nephritis[c]
	Membranoproliferative glomerular nephritis[c]
	Amyloid-type deposits
	Scleroderma renal crisis

The frequency of these manifestations is largely unknown as most are only case reports.
  [a] Common.
  [b] Uncommon.
  [c] Vary rare.

scleroderma overlapping with dermatomyositis, whose uninvolved skin biopsies revealed a particulate or speckled nuclear staining with specificity for IgG. The patients did well with corticosteroid treatment. Morphea has also been described in MCTD. A 19-year-old woman with morphea and a positive anti-RNP had speckled nuclear Ig immunofluorescence in the dermis of the morphea and was diagnosed with MCTD [47]. Generalized calcinosis can also occur in MCTD [48]. Some manifestations of skin involvement are given in Table 4.

There is one report of urticarial vasculitis occurring in a patient with MCTD [49]. Complements were normal in this patient. Angioedema and urticaria were the cutaneous manifestations.

Renal involvement

Renal involvement in MCTD can occur. Manifestations can include glomerulonephritis (GN), nephrotic syndrome, scleroderma renal crisis, amyloidosis, and renal infarcts. In one review [50], 11 of 30 patients who had MCTD had renal involvement; five patients had membranous GN, two patients had mesangial GN, one patient had mixed findings, and one patient had a sclerodermalike pattern on renal biopsy. Nine of 11 patients had nephrotic range proteinuria. Patients who have renal disease in MCTD have more systemic manifestations than those without. Treatment seemed to be successful: 72% of the patients who had nephritis and 62% of patients who were nephrotic experienced resolution or improvement with steroid treatment. Complement levels were not helpful in predicting who would have renal involvement [50]. Electron microscopic findings have revealed electron-dense deposits in the glomeruli compatible with immune complex deposition [51]. Another patient who had MCTD and nephrotic syndrome was found to have amyloid-type deposits that were larger than typical amyloid fibrils [52]. The significance of the larger deposits was not known.

An autopsy series of 25 patients who had MCTD was performed [53]. Sixteen subjects had renal dysfunction. Forty percent had membranous lesions, 7% had membranoproliferative, and some subjects had mesangial proliferative lesions. There was also intimal thickening in many renal arteries of these patients, such as that which is seen in scleroderma [53].

Anticardiolipin antibody syndrome can cause renal infarcts. This has been reported in one patient who had MCTD [54]. The patient improved with low-dose aspirin. Scleroderma renal crisis is recognized rarely in MCTD, and treatment with angiotensin-converting enzyme inhibitors, and occasionally prostacyclin analogs, may be indicated (see Table 4) [55].

Cardiac involvement in mixed connective tissue disease

The heart and surrounding structures can be involved in patients who have MCTD. Pericardial involvement is often underdiagnosed. Cardiomyopathy and valvular changes can also occur. Dropinski [56] characterized the cardiac manifestations of patients who had autoimmune diseases, including nine patients who had MCTD. It has been estimated that pericardial involvement occurs in 30% of patients who have MCTD, compared with 59% of patients who have scleroderma and 44% of patients who have SLE. It is less common in RA (24%) and polymyositis (11%). Rarely, cardiac tamponade has been observed in MCTD-related pericardial effusions [57]. Another case series described one patient who had MCTD who had angina and another patient who had pericardial effusion [58].

Cardiovascular autonomic dysfunction occurred in several patients who had MCTD and esophageal dysmotility [23]. Another patient with normal coronary arteries had pan-conduction cardiac defects with a right bundle branch block and primary AV block in association with MCTD and concomitant Sjögren's syndrome [59].

Thrombocytopenia purpura

Thrombotic TTP occurs in SLE. There are also several case reports in which it has been associated with MCTD [60–65]. TTP can be lethal in MCTD [61,63]. TTP is accompanied by a widespread vasculopathy with intimal proliferation and minimal fibrosis. Treatment has included cyclophosphamide, plasmapheresis, and plasma exchange [64].

Hematologic manifestations

Cytopenias, including thrombocytopenia, hemolytic anemia, anemia of chronic disease, and leukopenia, occur in MCTD. There are many case reports of severe thrombocytopenia in MCTD [66–69]. One patient who had hemolytic anemia also had TTP and was successfully treated with vincristine after failing prednisone, fresh frozen plasma, and prostacyclin therapy [69]. Thrombocytopenia results from the destruction of platelets coated with IgG autoantibodies, similar to that found in SLE [70]. Dessein [71] described a 49-year-old woman who had MCTD with antiphospholipid syndrome and severe immune thrombocytopenia. This patient developed skin infarctions. The low platelets and skin infarctions responded to immunosuppressive agents.

Pure red cell aplasia has been described in MCTD [72], although autoimmune hemolytic anemia is more common. Table 4 lists some hematologic manifestations.

Antiphospholipid antibodies in mixed connective tissue disease

Antiphospholipid syndrome is well described in SLE, including arterial or venous thrombosis and recurrent fetal loss. In one study [73], 15% of patients who had MCTD (7 of 48) had positive anticardiolipin antibodies, compared with 41% (24 of 59) of patients who had lupus. In a series of 28 patients who had MCTD (18% of whom had anticardiolipin antibodies), it was suggested that anticardiolipin antibodies correlated with thrombocytopenia but not with recurrent thrombosis or recurrent abortions [74]. However, classic antiphospholipid syndrome can occur in MCTD and can be fatal [75,76]. Unlike lupus, most anticardiolipin antibodies in MCTD have been β2 glycoprotein independent [77]. This could perhaps explain why some of the patients are less apt to clot or have full-blown antiphospholipid syndrome in MCTD (see Table 4).

Other autoimmune conditions in mixed connective tissue disease

Some patients with MCTD also have diabetes mellitus, autoimmune thyroiditis, and vitiligo gravis. Several case reports have demonstrated myasthenia gravis concomitantly with MCTD [78–80]. The association of MCTD with myasthenia gravis may be accompanied by Sjögren's syndrome, but this is rare [79,80].

Summary

There is a predilection for multiple different organ involvement in MCTD, including the heart, lung, kidney, muscle, joints, and skin. Thrombocytopenia is immune mediated and may be accompanied by anticardiolipin antibody syndrome or as part of TTP. Inflammatory arthritis is common and is frequently associated with damage, so treatment is required. Esophageal dysmotility is also common and requires frequent treatment. Vigilance is required in following patients who have MCTD to appropriately diagnose and treat frequent and rare manifestations of this multifaceted illness.

References

[1] Bennett RM, O'Connell DJ. The arthritis of mixed connective tissue disease. Ann Rheum Dis 1978;37:397–403.
[2] Ramos-Niembro F, Alarcon-Segovia D, Hernandez-Ortiz J. Articular manifestations of mixed connective tissue disease. Arthritis Rheum 1979;22:43–51.
[3] Halla JT, Hardin JG. Clinical features of the arthritis of mixed connective tissue disease. Arthritis Rheum 1978;21:497–503.
[4] O'Connell DJ, Bennett RM. Mixed connective tissue disease: clinical and radiological aspects of 20 cases. Br J Radiol 1977;50:620–5.
[5] Udoff EJ, Genant HK, Kozin F, et al. Mixed connective tissue disease: the spectrum radiographic manifestations. Radiology 1977;124:613–8.
[6] Piette JC, Le Thi HD, Ziza JM, et al. Jaccoud's rheumatism in Sharp's syndrome. Rev Rhum Mal Osteoartic 1988;55:153–4.

[7] Catoggio LJ, Evison G, Harkness JA, et al. The arthropathy of systemic sclerosis (scleroderma compared with mixed connective tissue disease. Clin Exp Rheumatol 1983;1:101–12.

[8] Alarcon-Segovia D, Uribe-Uribe O. Mutilans-like arthropathy in mixed connective tissue disease. Arthritis Rheum 1979;22:1013–8.

[9] Stuart RA, Maddison PJ. Atlantoaxial subluxation in a patient with mixed connective tissue disease. J Rheumatol 1991;18:1617–20.

[10] Huang CM. Gouty arthritis in a female patient with mixed connective tissue disease. Clin Rheumatol 2000;19:67–9.

[11] Hutton CW, Maddison PJ, Collins AJ, et al. Intra-articular apatite deposition in mixed connective tissue disease: crystallographic and technetium scanning characteristics. Ann Rheum Dis 1988;47:1027–30.

[12] Brandt J, Maier T, Rudwaleit M, et al. Co-occurrence of spondyloarthropathy and connective tissue disease: development of Sjogren's syndrome and mixed connective tissue disease (MCTD) in a patient with ankylosing spondylitis. Clin Exp Rheumatol 2002;20:80–4.

[13] Lanigan DT, Myall RW, West RA, et al. Condylysis in a patient with a mixed collagen vascular disease. Oral Surg Oral Med Oral Pathol 1979;48:198–204.

[14] Takei S, Maeno N, Shigemori M, et al. Two cases with SLE and MCTD developed after a long period of chronic arthritis that was initially diagnosed as JRA. Ryumachi 1997;37:702–8.

[15] Piirainen HI. Patients with arthritis and anti-U1-RNP antibodies: a 10-year follow-up. Br J Rheumatol 1990;29:345–8.

[16] Norman DA, Fleischmann RM. Gastrointestinal systemic sclerosis in serologic mixed connective tissue disease. Arthritis Rheum 1978;21:811–9.

[17] Tsianos EB, Drosos AA, Chiras CD, et al. Esophageal manometric findings in autoimmune rheumatic diseases: is scleroderma esophagus a specific entity? Rheumatol Int 1987;7:23–7.

[18] Marshall JB, Kretschmar JM, Gerhardt DC, et al. Gastrointestinal manifestations of mixed connective tissue disease. Gastroenterology 1990;98:1232–8.

[19] Doria A, Bonavina L, Anselmino M, et al. Esophageal involvement in mixed connective tissue disease. J Rheumatol 1991;18:685–90.

[20] Gutierrez F, Valenzuela JE, Ehresmann GR, et al. Esophageal dysfunction in patients with mixed connective tissue diseases and systemic lupus erythematosus. Dig Dis Sci 1982;27:592–7.

[21] Lapadula G, Muolo P, Semeraro F, et al. Esophageal motility disorders in the rheumatic diseases: a review of 150 patients. Clin Exp Rheumatol 1994;12:515–21.

[22] Dantas RO, Villanova MG, de Godoy RA. Esophageal dysfunction in patients with progressive systemic sclerosis and mixed connective tissue diseases. Arq Gastroenterol 1985;22:122–6.

[23] Stacher G, Merio R, Budka C, et al. Cardiovascular autonomic function, autoantibodies, and esophageal motor activity in patients with systemic sclerosis and mixed connective tissue disease. J Rheumatol 2000;27:692–7.

[24] Weber P, Ganser G, Frosch M, et al. Twenty-four hour intraesophageal pH monitoring in children and adolescents with scleroderma and mixed connective tissue disease. J Rheumatol 2000; 27:2692–5.

[25] Weston S, Thumshirn M, Wiste J, et al. Clinical and upper gastrointestinal motility features in systemic sclerosis and related disorders. Am J Gastroenterol 1998;93:1085–9.

[26] Matsumoto T, Kobayashi S, Shimizu H, et al. The liver in collagen diseases: pathologic study of 160 cases with particular reference to hepatic arteritis, primary biliary cirrhosis, autoimmune hepatitis and nodular regenerative hyperplasia of the liver. Liver 2000;20:366–73.

[27] Kmieciak Le Corguille M, Rocher P, Eugene C, et al. Autoimmune hepatitis, acute pancreatitis, mixed connective tissue disease and Sjogren's syndrome: a case report. Gastroenterol Clin Biol 2003;27:840–1.

[28] Hirose W, Nakane H, Misumi J, et al. Duodenal hemorrhage and dermal vasculitis associated with mixed connective tissue disease. J Rheumatol 1993;20:151–4.

[29] Lynn JT, Gossen G, Miller A, et al. Pneumatosis intestinalis in mixed connective tissue disease: two case reports and literature review. Arthritis Rheum 1984;27:1186–9.

[30] Goulet JR, Hurtubise M, Senecal JL. Retropneumoperitoneum and pneumatosis intestinalis in

2 patients with mixed connective tissue disease and the overlap syndrome. Clin Exp Rheumatol 1988;6:81–5.

[31] Nosho K, Takahashi H, Ikeda Y, et al. a case of protein-losing gastroenteropathy in association with mixed connective tissue disease which was successfully treated with cyclophosphamide pulse therapy. Ryumachi 1998;38:818–24.

[32] Showji Y, Nozawa R, Sato K, et al. Seroprevalence of heliobacter pylori infection in patients with connective tissue diseases. Microbiol Immunol 1996;40:499–503.

[33] Sharp GC. Mixed connective tissue disease. Bull Rheum Dis 1975;25:828–31.

[34] Setty YN, Pittman CB, Mahale AS, et al. Sicca symptoms and anti-SSA/Ro antibodies are common in mixed connective tissue disease. J Rheumatol 2002;29:487–9.

[35] Helenius LM, Hietanen JH, Helenius I, et al. Focal sialadenitis in patients with ankylosing spondylitis and spondyloarthropathy: a comparison with patients with rheumatoid arthritis or mixed connective tissue disease. Ann Rheum Dis 2001;60:744–9.

[36] Alarcon-Segovia D. Symptomatic Sjogren's syndrome in mixed connective tissue disease. J Rheumatol 1976;3:191–5.

[37] Konttinen YT, Tuominen TS, Piirainen HI, et al. Signs and symptoms in the masticatory system in ten patients with mixed connective tissue disease. Scand J Rheumatol 1990;19:363–73.

[38] Alfaor-Giner A, Penarrocha-Diago M, Bagan-Sebastian JV. Orofacial manifestations of mixed connective tissue disease with an uncommon serologic evolution. Oral Surg Oral Med Oral Pathol 1992;73:441–4.

[39] Wada T, Motoo Y, Ohmizo R, et al. Association of mixed connective tissue disease, Sjogren's syndrome and autoimmune hepatitis: report of a case. Jpn J Med 1991;30:278–80.

[40] Min JK, Han NI, Kim JA, et al. A case of cholestatic autoimmune hepatitis and liver failure: an unusual hepatic manifestation in mixed connective tissue disease and Sjogren's syndrome. J Korean Med Sci 2001;16:512–5.

[41] Frayha RA, Nasr FW, Mufarrij AA. Mixed connective tissue disease, Sjogren's syndrome and abdominal pseudolymphoma. Br J Rheumatol 1985;24:70–3.

[42] Hameenkorpi R, Ruuska P, Forsberg S, et al. More evidence of distinctive features of mixed connective tissue disease. Scand J Rheumatol 1993;22:63–8.

[43] Oh YB, Jun JB, Kim CK, et al. Mixed connective tissue disease associated with skin defects of livedoid vasculitis. Clin Rheumatol 2000;19:381–4.

[44] Magro CM, Crowson AN, Regauer S. Mixed connective tissue disease: a clinical, histologic and immunofluorescence study of eight cases. Am J Dermatopathol 1997;19:206–13.

[45] Gilliam JN, Prystowsky SD. Conversion of discoid lupus erythematosus to mixed connective tissue disease. J Rheumatol 1977;4:165–9.

[46] Bentley-Phillips CB, Geake TM. Mixed connective tissue disease characterized by speckled epidermal nuclear IgG depostion in the skin. Br J Dermatol 1980;102:529–33.

[47] Golding DN. Morphoea (localized scleroderma) in a patient with mixed connective tissue disease. Ann Rheum Dis 1986;45:523–5.

[48] Baurle G, Hornstein OP. Generalized cutaneous calcinosis and mixed connective tissue disease. Dermatologica 1979;158:257–68.

[49] Asherson RA, D'Cruz D, Stephens CJ, et al. Urticarial vasculitis in a connective tissue disease clinic: patterns, presentations, and treatment. Semin Arthritis Rheum 1991;20:285–96.

[50] Kitridou RC, Akmal M, Turkel SB, et al. Renal involvement in mixed connective tissue disease: a longitudinal clinicopathologic study. Semin Arthritis Rheum 1986;16:135–45.

[51] Kobayashi S, Nagase M, Kimura M, et al. Renal involvement in mixed connective tissue disease: report of 5 cases. Am J Nephrol 1985;5:282–9.

[52] Kessler E, Halpern M, Chagnac A, et al. Unusual renal deposit in mixed connective tissue disease. Arch Pathol Lab Med 1992;116:261–4.

[53] Sawai T, Murakami K, Kurasono Y. Morphometric analysis of the kidney lesions in mixed connective tissue disease (MCTD). Tohoku J Exp Med 1994;174:141–54.

[54] Perinbasekar S, Chawla K, Rosner F, et al. Complete recovery from renal infarcts in a patient with mixed connective tissue disease. Am J Kidney Dis 1995;26:649–53.

[55] Satoh K, Imai H, Yasuda T, et al. Scleroderma renal crisis in a patient with mixed connective tissue disease. Am J Kidney Dis 1994;24:215–8.

[56] Dropinski J, Szczeklik W, Rubis P. Cardiac involvement is systemic autoimmune disease. Pol Arch Med Wewn 2003;109:375–81.

[57] Langley RL, Treadwell EL. Cardiac tamponade and pericardial disorders in connective tissue diseases: case report and literature review. J Natl Med Assoc 1994;86:149–53.

[58] Dutschmann L, Ferreira C, De Sousa G, et al. Cardiac manifestations of connective tissue diseases. Acta Med Port 1989;2:103–10.

[59] Rakovec P, Kenda MF, Rozman B, et al. Panconductional defect in mixed connective tissue disease: association with Sjogren's syndrome. Chest 1982;81:257–9.

[60] Paice EW, Smaith ML. Thrombotic thrombocytopenic purpura occurrence in a patient with mixed connective tissue disease. Rheumatol Int 1984;4:141–2.

[61] Bodolay E, Gaal J, Vegh J, et al. Evaluation of survival in mixed connective tissue disease (MCTD). Orv Hetil 2002;143:2543–8.

[62] Baron BW, Martin MS, Sucharetza BS, et al. Four patients with both thrombotic thrombocytopenic purpura and autoimmune thrombocytopenic purpura: the concept of a mixed immune thrombocytopenia syndrome and indications for plasma exchange. J Clin Apheresis 2001;16:179–85.

[63] Kato A, Suzuki Y, Fujigaki Y, et al. Thrombotic thrombocytopenic purpura associated with mixed connective tissue disease. Rheumatol Int 2002;22:122–5.

[64] Braun J, Sieper J, Schwarz A, et al. Widespread vasculopathy with hemolytic uremic syndrome, perimyocarditis and cystic pancreatitis in a young woman with mixed connective tissue disease: case report and review of the literature. Rheumatol Int 1993;13:31–6.

[65] Poullin P, Lefevre P, Durand JM. Mixed connective tissue disease with hemolytic anemia and severe thrombocytopenia due to thrombotic thrombocytopenic purpura. Am J Hematol 1999; 61:275.

[66] de Rooij DJ, van de Putte LB, van Beusekom HJ. Severe thrombocytopenia in mixed connective tissue disease. Scand J Rheumatol 1982;11:184–6.

[67] Segond P, Yeni P, Jacquot JM, et al. Severe autoimmune anemia and thrombopenia in mixed connective tissue disease. Arthritis Rheum 1978;21:995–7.

[68] Richart C, Pujol-Borrell R. Autoimmune hemolytic anemia and idiopathic thrombocytopenia purpura preceding a mixed connective tissue disease. Med Clin (Barc) 1983;81:370.

[69] ter Borg EJ, Houtman PM, Kallenberg CG, et al. Thrombocytopenia and hemolytic anemia in a patient with mixed connective tissue disease due to thrombotic thrombocytopenic purpura. J Rheumatol 1988;15:1174–7.

[70] Shimizu Y, Nojima Y, Mori M. Increased levels of platelet-associated immunoglobin G in a patient with mixed connective tissue disease. Hong Kong Med J 2002;8:285–7.

[71] Dessein PH, Lamparelli RD, Phillips SA, et al. Severe immune thrombocytopenia and the development of skin infarctions in a patient with an overlap syndrome. J Rheumatol 1989; 16:1494–6.

[72] Julkunen H, Jantti J, Pettersson T. Pure red cell aplasia in mixed connective tissue disease. J Rheumatol 1989;16:1385–6.

[73] Komatireddy GR, Wang GS, Sharp GC, et al. Antiphospholipid antibodies among anti-U1-70 kDa autoantibody positive patients with mixed connective tissue disease. J Rheumatol 1997;24: 319–22.

[74] Doria A, Ruffatti A, Calligaro A, et al. Antiphospholipid antibodies in mixed connective tissue disease. Clin Rheumatol 1992;11:48–50.

[75] Zuber M, Krazhofer N, Lindemuth R, et al. A patient with mixed collagen disease, antiphospholipid syndrome and Sjogren's syndrome. Med Klin 1998;93:34–8.

[76] Gluck T, Muller-Ladner U, Speicher A, et al. Fatal sinus vein thrombosis in a patient with mixed connective tissue disease and secondary antiphospholipid antibody syndrome. Med Klin 2001; 96:361–4.

[77] Mendonca LL, Amengual O, Atsumi T, et al. Most anticardiolipin antibodies in mixed connective tissue disease are beta2-glycoprotein independent. J Rheumatol 1998;25:189–90.

[78] Johannson EA, Niemi KM, Lassus A, et al. Mixed connective tissue disease: a follow-up study of 12 patients with special reference to cold sensitivity and skin manifestations. Acta Derm Venereol 1981;61:225–31.
[79] Yasuda M, Nobunaga M. The association of myasthenia gravis and connective tissue diseases: the role of Sjogren's syndrome. Fukuoka Igaku Zasshi 1994;85:38–51.
[80] Yasuda M, Loo M, Shiokawa S, et al. Mixed connective tissue disease presenting myasthenia gravis. Intern Med 1993;32:633–7.

ELSEVIER
SAUNDERS

RHEUMATIC
DISEASE CLINICS
OF NORTH AMERICA

Rheum Dis Clin N Am 31 (2005) 535–547

The Prognosis of Mixed Connective Tissue Disease

Ingrid E. Lundberg, MD, PhD

*Rheumatology Unit, Department of Medicine, Karolinska University Hospital, Solna,
Karolinska Institutet, SE-171 76 Stockholm, Sweden*

Mixed connective tissue disease (MCTD) was first described in 1972 as an entity with mixed features of systemic lupus erythematosus (SLE), systemic sclerosis, and polymyositis together with the presence of high-titer antinuclear antibodies and high-titer antiribonucleoprotein (anti-RNP) antibodies [1]. Later, significant arthritis that resembled rheumatoid arthritis (RA) was reported as a frequent finding in patients who had MCTD [2–4]. In the first description of the clinical phenotype of MCTD, the absence of serious renal involvement was reported as a characteristic feature of these patients, in contrast with patients who have SLE. Furthermore, a striking response to corticosteroid therapy was reported [1]. This overall favorable prognosis was questioned in a follow-up of this first case-series of patients who had MCTD [4,5]. Since these first contradictory reports on prognosis in patients who had MCTD, a few more reports on long-term prognosis have been published. These reports are summarized in this article; however, epidemiologic studies that include long-term follow-up of patients who have MCTD characteristics are scarce and include only a limited number of patients because of the rarity of this condition. Moreover, epidemiologic studies on outcome and prognosis that include

This work was supported by the Swedish Rheumatism Association. The author has received unrestricted research grants from Schering Plough and Baxter, an honorarium from Pfizer for teaching courses that were organized by the Swedish Society for Rheumatology, and owns stock in pharmaceutical companies.

E-mail address: ingrid.lundberg@medks.ki.se

relevant control populations are missing. This makes the overall prognosis in MCTD uncertain.

The presence of anti-RNP bodies in high titers is the laboratory hallmark of MCTD [1,6]. It was demonstrated that these anti-RNP antibodies in patients who have MCTD constitute antibodies that are directed to U1 small nuclear ribonucleoprotein (snRNP) autoantigens. In patients who have MCTD, these autoantibodies have a high specificity for a U1–70-kd polypeptide [7]. In later reports, the autoantibodies in patients who have MCTD are referred to as anti-U1 snRNP autoantibodies or—when tested more specifically—as anti-U1–70-kd snRNP autoantibodies [5,7–10]. The term anti/U1 snRNP antibodies is used in this article unless more detailed information is available on the specificity of these autoantibodies.

Sequential clinical and laboratory features

MCTD evolves with time and patients who have MCTD typically develop new clinical and laboratory characteristics. This became evident from long-term follow-up studies of patients who had anti-U1 snRNP antibodies [5,9, 11,12]. Thus, at first presentation, patients who have anti-U1snRNP antibodies may display only one or a few organ manifestations in addition to positive anti-U1 snRNP antibodies; at that time point they may not fulfill the classification criteria for MCTD or any other defined connective tissue disease. If they do not fulfill classification criteria for another defined connective tissue disease they often are classified as having undifferentiated connective tissue disease (UCTD) [13]. Some patients who have anti-U1 snRNP antibodies may fulfill criteria for another defined disease, such as RA, SLE, systemic sclerosis, or polymyositis, at first evaluation and new organ manifestations may evolve with time. There also are patients who have anti-U1 snRNP antibodies who present with overlapping features.

Transition from a more limited disease to a disease with overlap features was observed frequently in patients who had anti-U1 snRNP with a mean follow-up of more than 10 years [5,11,14]. In one prospective study, 60% of the patients had clinical symptoms and signs that were compatible with one inflammatory connective tissue disease at presentation and up to 1 to 2 years after their first medical evaluation; however, after a mean follow-up of 6 years, 90% fulfilled the criteria for MCTD [5]. A similar development of new clinical manifestations was observed in a prospective study of 32 patients who had anti-U1 snRNP antibodies. In this study, only 35% of the patients fulfilled the criteria for any defined connective tissue disease at first evaluation; 3 fulfilled the criteria for MCTD [1] and 18 were classified as having UCTD. After a mean observation time of 6 years, the diagnosis was changed in 53% (17 cases) of the patients. Of the 18 patients who had UCTD, 15 developed symptoms or signs that were compatible with a defined diagnosis: 11 had MCTD, 2 developed SLE, and

2 fulfilled the criteria for MCTD and SLE [11]. In a study of 46 patients who had anti-U1snRNP antibodies with a minimal follow-up of 5 years, 33 were classified initially as having MCTD, 10 as having SLE, 2 as having RA, and 1 as having systemic sclerosis. After a mean follow-up time of 15 ± 6 years, development of new clinical symptoms were common; 22 of the 46 patients fulfilled the criteria for another defined inflammatory connective tissue disease. Thus, 55% of those who initially were diagnosed with MCTD also fulfilled the criteria of at least one more rheumatic disease, most often systemic sclerosis or SLE. Of the 10 patients who were diagnosed initially as having SLE, 4 developed clinical manifestations that were compatible with systemic sclerosis [14].

The long-term development of MCTD may vary. From long-term follow up studies, it can be concluded that MCTD may develop into a mild disease with benign prognosis or patients may develop a serious disease with vascular changes that are dominated by pulmonary hypertension and increased mortality [4,15]. In the most comprehensive evaluation of long-term outcome (a mean observation of 15 years) in 47 patients who had MCTD, 17 patients were classified as being in remission (defined as a prednisone dose of less than 6 mg/d and no cytotoxic therapy), 12 were improved but received prednisolone (6–19 mg/d), 7 had persistently active disease, and 11 patients were deceased [15]. Of those who died, most had active disease and had undergone aggressive treatment, and pulmonary hypertension was frequent in this group (7 of 11; 64%) compared with the remainder (4 of 36; 11%). Only two of those who died were in remission before their deaths. They died from a cerebrovascular accident or a malignancy. Clinical remission was accompanied by a significant reduction of anti-U1 snRNP antibody titers, in contrast to those who had persisting active disease and whose autoantibody levels were consistently high. In most patients who were in remission, anti-U1 snRNP antibodies were not detectable. In another long-term follow-up study, clinical and serologic data were related to serum levels of the cytokines, interleukin-10 and tumor necrosis factor, in a series of serum samples that were collected over 2 to 11 years [12]. Also, in this study, the disease activity was greater during the first years after disease onset and decreased with time. This clinical evolution was accompanied by a decrease of serum levels of anti-U1 snRNP antibodies.

From long-term follow-up studies, we can conclude that approximately one third of patients who have MCTD have a benign course and go into remission, and one third have a more aggressive course with less favorable response to treatment. Approximately one third of patients who have MCTD improved with immunosuppressive treatment but still required immunosuppressive therapy after several years. The worst prognosis with a high mortality was associated with the presence of pulmonary hypertension, which must be regarded as the most serious complication in MCTD. In one prospective study, 23% of patients who had MCTD developed pulmonary hypertension [15]. Concurrence of MCTD and IgG anticardiolipin antibodies (aCL) correlated significantly with pulmonary hypertension, although those patients did not have any other thromboembolic manifestations of the antiphospholipid syndrome.

Mortality

Long-term follow up studies on mortality in patients who have MCTD are few and often include a limited number of patients, which reflects the rarity of this condition (Table 1). In five series of MCTD with a total of 194 patients, the mortality generally was low (mean, 13%; range, 4–35%) in patients who had a disease duration of 6 to 12 years [4,8,9,16,17]. These data are from tertiary referral centers, and therefore, may include some patients who were more severely ill. In a prospective study of 34 patients with a mean disease duration of 6 to 12 years, the mortality was 12% [5]. In the most comprehensive and most recent longitudinal study of long-term outcome in patients who had MCTD, 47 patients were followed for a mean of 15 years (range, 3 to 29 years) [15]. The mortality in this study was 23%.

Based on a 1997 review of the literature that summarized 30 reports, the mortality in children was 7.6% [18]. The mortality in different reports varied between 3.9% and 27%. These data are comparable to the mortality in juvenile SLE (4.8%) and juvenile systemic sclerosis (5.3%) [18].

Comparison data of mortality with population-matched controls are missing for patients who have MCTD. Because MCTD affects young individuals (mean age at onset, 28–37 years) with a strong predominance in women (84%) [5,8,15], even a 13% mortality after a disease duration of 6 to 12 years indicates a greatly enhanced risk of premature death.

Cause of death

The predominating causes of death in patients who have MCTD are pulmonary hypertension, associated with proliferative vascular disease, and severe infections [5,15]. In a retrospective study of 23 patients who had clinical and

Table 1
Mortality rate in patients who have mixed connective tissue disease

First author, year [Ref.]	No. of patients	Disease duration (y)	No. of deaths (mortality rate in %)
Sharp, 1976 [8]	100	6	4 (4)
Singsen, 1977 [17][a]	15	6.8	4 (27)
Nimelstein, 1980 [4]	22	12	8 (36)
Bennett, 1980 [20]	20	5 (follow-up)	4 (20)
Grant, 1981 [9]	23	8.3 (follow-up)	5 (22)
Sullivan, 1984 [5]	34	11	4 (12)
Piirainen, 1990 [3]	23	17	5 (22)
Michels, 1997 [18][a]	33	7.6	2 (6)
Burdt, 1999 [15]	47	15 (follow-up)	11 (23)
Total	**317**		**47 (15)**

[a] Juvenile cases.

serologic features of MCTD, 5 patients had died at the time of study [9]. This cohort included 2 individuals who were younger than 20 years and 3 patients who were older than 60 years. Pulmonary disease, pulmonary hypertension, and congestive heart failure were the cause of death in four of five cases. These 4 patients had laboratory evidence of active MCTD. One died from squamous cell carcinoma of the lung, which was regarded as being unrelated to the MCTD [9].

In a more recent long-term follow-up study of adults who had MCTD, pulmonary hypertension was the cause of death or contributed to severe illness in 9 of the 11 patients who died [15]. The autopsy findings in patients who had MCTD and pulmonary hypertension were dominated by proliferative vascular changes in the lungs, endomyocardial vessels, and intrarenal vessels. This was in contrast to minimal signs of interstitial fibrosis. These observations support the notion of a proliferative vascular process, rather than interstitial lung disease as the disease mechanisms in MCTD, at least in patients who develop pulmonary hypertension.

In contrast to SLE, premature death that is due to cardiovascular disease, but not attributable to pulmonary hypertension, was reported rarely in patients who had MCTD. In a few cases, significant myocarditis preceded death that was due to heart failure [20]. Increased mortality that is caused by premature atherosclerosis has not been reported in MCTD.

Severe infection is the second most commonly reported cause of death in adult patients who have MCTD; this contributed to death in 6 of 11 patients in one study [15]. The reported infections were bacterial infections, such as septicemia, pneumonia, and peritonitis.

In children who had MCTD, the most common cause of death was severe infection that often was related to immunosuppressive treatment [18]. Other reported causes of death in children are cerebral complications, pulmonary hypertension, and heart-failure that is associated with myocarditis. In children, there also are reports of death that is related to renal disease (hemolytic uremic syndrome or glomerulonephritis).

Morbidity

The data on long-term morbidity in patients who have MCTD in relation to prognosis also are limited. The long-term outcome varies from remission to progressive inflammatory active disease. In most cases, features of inflammation seem to vanish or diminish [12,15]. The frequency of Raynaud's phenomenon and esophageal hypomotility also was reduced in a long-term follow-up study, whereas sclerodactyly or diffuse sclerosis, pulmonary dysfunction, pulmonary hypertension, and nervous system disease persisted [15]. Although signs of active arthritis were a less common clinical symptom among patients who had a late phase of MCTD when compared with an early phase, 40% still had problems with arthralgia or arthritis after a mean disease duration of more than 15 years [15]. In another long-term follow-up study of patients who had MCTD, persistent morbidity was reported from arthritis, easy fatiguability, and dyspnea on exertion [19]. Although many patients who have MCTD go into remission with low inflammatory disease activity, they still may have functional impairment that is due to organ damage.

Joints

The joints are affected frequently in patients who have MCTD, and various features are present. Common joint symptoms include arthralgia and arthritis; they often are among the first symptoms of disease. The arthritis can be mono-, oligo-, or polyarticular rheumatoid arthritis-like with a symmetric distribution of small joints [3,21]. The most frequently reported radiologic features of bone and joints are periarticular, marginal bone erosions in 40% to 70% of patients who have MCTD [2,3,22–24]. Other characteristic radiologic features are erosions in the tufts of the distal phalanges of the fingers and avascular necrosis [2,22]. Joint space narrowing and generalized osteopenia are less common findings [22]. The bone erosions are located mainly in the wrists and interphalangeal and metacarpal-phalangeal joints of the hands, and, less often, the feet. The severity of arthritis varies. In most patients who have anti-RNP antibodies, the erosions are small with an asymmetric distribution in scattered joints, even after several years of arthritis. After a mean disease duration of 10 years, only minor erosions were detected, although there are reports of occasional patients who have severe, destructive arthritis with bone resorptions that resemble the mutilans type of psoriatic arthritis [22]. In one study, the severity of the erosive disease in patients who had MCTD was correlated to the presence of rheumatoid factor [3], but this was not the case in another study [22]. Soft tissue calcifications that resemble those in patients who have systemic sclerosis were also reported [2,22].

Some patients develop joint deformities. The degree of impairment that is due to severe joint disease varies between studies. It is difficult to compare the functional outcome between different studies because there is no validated outcome measure for patients who have MCTD, and the outcome measures that were used vary between studies or are absent. Another explanation for the discrepancy between reports could be referral bias. Still, functional impairment that is due to joint disease seems to be higher in patient cohorts who have disease of longer duration [20]. It also is possible that functional impairment could be a consequence not only of erosive disease, but also of joint deformities resulting from periarticular, soft tissue involvement resembling Jaccoud's deformities that are sometimes seen in patients who have SLE. In one study, the arthritis was reported to be generally mild but most of the patients (12/20) had a functional disability of grade II/IV according to Steinbrocker's classification, 6 of 20 patients had a functional disability of grade III/IV, and only 2 were in class I with no impact on daily living [19]. From these studies, it can be concluded that arthritis is a major clinical problem in patients who have MCTD. It affects mainly small joints and it may be erosive, but generally with a slow progression; however, it still has an impact on daily function even after many years of disease.

Muscles

Myositis has been reported as a frequent manifestation in patients who have anti-U1 snRNP antibodies or MCTD. A favorable response to cortico-steroids in patients who had anti-U1snRNP antibodies and myositis was seen in one study [25]. In another study, no difference in response to immunosuppressive treatment was observed compared with other inflammatory myopathies [26]. Both of these reports are limited by a small number of patients and the absence of a standardized outcome measure of muscle function. Thus, more studies are needed to answer the question of prognosis in relation to the presence of myo-sitis in patients who have MCTD.

Lung involvement

Lung involvement with pulmonary hypertension was reported as the most serious clinical problem in a prospective study of 34 patients who had MCTD with a mean observation time of 6 years [5]. In several studies, pulmonary hypertension was associated with a poor prognosis and was a major cause of death in patients who had MCTD [5,15,27]. In one study, pulmonary hypertension was recorded in 65% of those who underwent cardiac catheteri-zation, regardless of clinical symptoms of the lungs [27]. There is no clinical or laboratory test to suggest pulmonary hypertension in patients who have MCTD. In comparison with other CTDs that are accompanied by pulmonary hyper-tension, patients who had MCTD had a quicker occurrence of pulmonary hypertension and a shorter survival; however, in other aspects there were no differences [28]. Although pulmonary hypertension is a major risk factor for death, the course of pulmonary hypertension is not always progressive and some patients improve with treatment [5,15,29]. There are no controlled clinical trials in patients who have MCTD, but there are a few reports which suggest improve-ment on pulmonary function tests after treatment with corticosteroids alone or in combination with cyclophosphamide, at least in some cases with pulmonary hypertension [5,15]. Objective improvement was seen rarely on chest radiograph, however [5]. Positive effect also was recorded in a few cases on pulmonary vascular resistance after treatment with oral nifedipine [29].

An increased knowledge of the pathogenic mechanisms that lead to pulmonary hypertension is needed to improve treatment and outcome of this fatal compli-cation in MCTD. The pathophysiology of pulmonary hypertension in patients who have MCTD mainly is related to vascular disease, and rarely, to pulmonary fibrosis. From autopsy studies it was demonstrated that pulmonary hypertension was associated with intimal proliferation of small pulmonary arteries and arterioles and smooth muscle hypertrophy with only sporadic lymphocytic infiltration in the lungs [27]. A similar finding of intimal proliferation was observed in the epicardial and intramural coronary arteries. It was hypothesized that pulmonary hypertension in MCTD was related to proliferative vascular abnormalities that involve small pulmonary vessels. The pathogenic mechanisms behind the vascular abnormalities still need to be clarified, however.

Cardiovascular disease

Epidemiologic studies of cardiac involvement in patients who have myositis and MCTD largely are lacking, which makes conclusions about the frequency and prognosis of clinical and subclinical cardiac manifestations uncertain. In the few published reports, the frequency of cardiac involvement in patients who had MCTD varied between 11% and 85%, depending on patient selection, and definitions of cardiac involvement, and methods used to detect cardiac manifestations [11,27,30]. In the study by Alpert and colleagues [27], in which a high prevalence of cardiac manifestations was reported, all patients were subject to investigations of cardiac involvement, regardless of symptoms. The most frequently detected cardiac manifestations were pericarditis in 29%, and mitral valve prolapse in 26%. There also were reports of myocarditis, conduction disturbances (including complete heart block), and abnormal left ventricular diastolic filling pattern [27,30]. Using echocardiography to detect cardiac abnormalities, right ventricular enlargement was more common than left ventricular enlargement. Clinically significant cardiac involvement is rare in patients who have MCTD. Most reported cases of myocarditis improved with corticosteroid treatment alone or in combination with azathioprine or cyclophosphamide. Despite initial improvement with immunosuppressive treatment there is a risk of relapse or later development of heart failure [19,31]. Other cardiovascular events, such as stroke, were reported rarely in MCTD [15].

Antiphospholipid antibodies which were detected as anticardiolipin antibodies were present in approximately 15% of patients who had MCTD; this is less frequent than in patients who had SLE [32,33]. When present, the anticardiolipin antibodies were not associated with thromboembolic events or other manifestations that are characteristic of the antiphospholipid syndrome. The explanation for the absence of clinical manifestations that are associated with antiphospholipid syndrome in other patients is uncertain, but might be explained by the low or medium elevated titers of IgG antibodies and the prevalent IgM isotype antibodies.

Digital ulcers

Raynaud's phenomenon is a common initial symptom in MCTD. It may be severe; in occasional patients it is associated with digital necrosis or gangrene of multiple finger tips [34,35]. The prognosis of Raynaud's phenomenon is not invariably poor because it may improve over time with a reduction in frequency [15].

Gastrointestinal involvement

Gastrointestinal symptoms are common and were reported in 66% to 74% of patients who had MCTD [15,36,37]. The most frequently reported symptoms result from esophageal involvement, such as heartburn in 48% and dysphagia in 38% [36]. Sensitive tests, such as esophageal manometry, also detected abnormal motility in asymptomatic patients which indicated an even more frequent involvement of this organ [20,37]. In comparison with systemic sclerosis, the morphologic and functional abnormalities of the esophageal involvement was less severe in patients who had MCTD [37]. There was no correlation between the degree of esophageal involvement and disease activity or scleroderma-like skin involvement [37]. In a small, open longitudinal study, improved esophageal function was determined by manometry after corticosteroid treatment for a mean duration of 67 weeks [36]. This is in contrast to the reported higher degree of impaired manometric findings with longer disease duration in another report [37]. In the latter study, the mean disease duration was longer— more than 120 months in patients who had greater impairment—and the esophageal function was not related to treatment. It can be concluded that the degree of esophageal hypomotility is reversible, at least in part, but a controlled trial is needed to determine whether the esophageal involvement is responsive to corticosteroid treatment.

Other parts of the gastrointestinal tract also may be affected in MCTD. Dilation of the small bowel with malabsorption that was due to bacterial overgrowth and colon diverticulosis were reported in occasional patients; however, it is not known whether this was more frequent than in a healthy population because no comparator group was included [20,36].

Renal involvement

The frequency of renal involvement varied between 5% and 36% in different cohorts of patients who had MCTD [8,38]. The most comprehensive histopathologic data of renal involvement comes from a longitudinal study in which 11 of 30 patients had clinically significant proteinuria [38]. The histopathology was dominated by mild mesangial changes and interstitial fibrosis. Active lesions with cellular crescents were detected in only 1 patient. Six patients were classified as having membranous nephropathy, 2 had mesangial glomerulitis, 1 had focal sclerosing glomerulonephritis, 1 had membranoproliferative nephritis, and 1 had focal proliferative glomerulonephritis and arteritis. After treatment with corticosteroids, 72% of nephropathy episodes resolved or were reduced substantially, and renal function remained normal in 58% of the patients. Chronic renal failure developed in 2 patients. In a summary of 76 published cases of MCTD with renal biopsies, the renal disease was classified as membranous nephropathy in 34%, as mesangial in 30%, and as proliferative glomerulonephritis in 17% [38]. Fourteen percent of these patients developed chronic renal failure. In the long-term follow-up study by Burdt and colleagues [15], 11% developed clinically significant renal disease—and at the last evaluation of their cohort—2% (1 patient) had signs of persistent renal disease. It is possible that the difference in renal involvement between the studies by Kitridou and colleagues [38] and Burdt and colleagues [15] can be explained by patient selection. One difference between these two studies was ethnic background; in the study by Kitridou and coworkers, 20 of the 30 patients were black, 8 were Hispanic, and 2 were white, whereas in the study by Burdt and coworkers, 38 of the 47 patients were white and 9 were black. Whether the different clinical profiles and outcome in patients who had MCTD could be related to ethnicity, different genetic background, or other factors is not known.

Osteoporosis

There is an increased risk for osteoporosis as a long-term consequence in other rheumatic diseases, in particular RA and SLE. There is only one report on osteoporosis in patients who had MCTD [39]. This included a report of bone mineral density of the lumbar spine and femoral neck in 58 postmenopausal women who had MCTD with a mean disease duration of 9.1 years (range, 1–16 years). In the lumbar spine, but not in the femoral neck, bone mineral density was decreased in 25.8% (T-score <-2.5). A low bone mineral density was associated with longer disease duration and corticosteroid therapy. Women who had MCTD also had lower serum levels of estradiol, testosterone, and dehydroepiandrosterone in comparison with controls; this indicates that low levels of sex hormones could contribute to osteoporosis in patients who have MCTD. These observations need to be confirmed in a larger study.

Summary

From long-term follow-up studies, it can be concluded that the prognosis for patients who have MCTD varies from a benign, long-term outcome with remission to a severe, progressive disease course. Approximately one third of patients who have MCTD have a benign course and go into remission, one third have an aggressive course, and one third have a partial response with immunosuppressive treatment but still require immunosuppressive therapy after several years. The worst prognosis with a high mortality is associated with the presence of pulmonary hypertension, which must be regarded as the most serious complication in MCTD. The frequency of pulmonary hypertension in MCTD is uncertain but was 23% in one study and correlated with the presence of IgG aCL. Pulmonary hypertension is associated with proliferative vascular abnormalities that involve small pulmonary vessels, rather than interstitial lung disease. Long-term morbidity is affected by the presence of pulmonary hypertension and by impairment that results from arthritis and general fatigue.

Acknowledgments

The author is grateful to Associate Professor Ronald van Vollenhoven for linguistic advice.

References

[1] Sharp GC, Irvin WS, Tan EM, et al. Mixed connective tissue disease—an apparently distinct rheumatic disease syndrome associated with a specific antibody to an extractable nuclear antigen(ENA). Am J Med 1972;52(2):148–59.

[2] Silver TM, Farber SJ, Bole GG, et al. Radiological features of mixed connective tissue disease and scleroderma–systemic lupus erythematosus overlap. Radiology 1976;120(2):269–75.

[3] Piirainen HI. Patients with arthritis and anti U1-RNP antibodies: a 10-year follow up. Br J Rheumatol 1990;29:345–8.

[4] Nimelstein SH, Brody S, McShane D, et al. Mixed connective tissue disease: a subsequent evaluation of the original 25 patients. Medicine (Baltimore) 1980;59(4):239–48.

[5] Sullivan WD, Hurst DJ, Harmon CE, et al. A prospective evaluation emphasizing pulmonary involvement in patients with mixed connective tissue disease. Medicine (Baltimore) 1984;63(2): 92–107.

[6] Sharp GC, Irvin WS, LaRoque RL, et al. Association of autoantibodies to different nuclear antigens with clinical patterns of rheumatic disease and responsiveness to therapy. J Clin Invest 1971;50(2):350–9.

[7] Pettersson I, Wang G, Smith EI, et al. The use of immunoblotting and immunoprecipitation of (U) small nuclear ribonucleoproteins in the analysis of sera of patients with mixed connective tissue disease and systemic lupus erythematosus. A cross-sectional, longitudinal study. Arthritis Rheum 1986;29(8):986–96.

[8] Sharp GC, Irvin WS, May CM, et al. Association of antibodies to ribonucleoprotein and Sm antigens with mixed connective-tissue disease, systematic lupus erythematosus and other rheumatic diseases. N Engl J Med 1976;295(21):1149–54.

[9] Grant KD, Adams LE, Hess EV. Mixed connective tissue disease - a subset with sequential clinical and laboratory features. J Rheumatol 1981;8(4):587–98.

[10] Sharp GC. MCTD: a concept which stood the test of time. Lupus 2002;11(6):333–9.

[11] Lundberg I, Hedfors E. Clinical course of patients with anti-RNP antibodies. A prospective study of 32 patients. J Rheumatol 1991;18(10):1511–9.

[12] Hassan AB, Gunnarsson I, Karlsson G, et al. Longitudinal study of interleukin-10, tumor necrosis factor-alpha, anti-U1-snRNP antibody levels and disease activity in patients with mixed connective tissue disease. Scand J Rheumatol 2001;30(5):282–9.

[13] Pestelli E, Volpi W, Giomi B, et al. Undifferentiated connective tissue disease and its cutaneous manifestations. J Eur Acad Dermatol Venereol 2003;17:715–7.

[14] van den Hoogen FH, Spronk PE, Boerbooms AM, et al. Long-term follow-up of 46 patients with anti-(U1)snRNP antibodies. Br J Rheumatol 1994;33(12):1117–20.

[15] Burdt MA, Hoffman RW, Deutscher SL, et al. Long-term outcome in mixed connective tissue disease: longitudinal clinical and serologic findings. Arthritis Rheum 1999;42(5):899–909.

[16] Sharp GC. Diagnostic criteria for classification of MCTD and therapy and prognosis of MCTD. In: Sharp GC, Kasukawa R, editors. Mixed connective tissue disease and anti-nuclear antibodies. Amsterdam: Elsevier; 1987. p. 315–24.

[17] Singsen BH, Bernstein BH, Kornreich HK, et al. Mixed connective tissue disease in childhood. A clinical and serologic survey. J Pediatr 1977;90(6):893–900.

[18] Michels H. Course of mixed connective tissue disease in children. Ann Med 1997;29(5):359–64.

[19] Bennett RM, O'Connell DJ. Mixed connective tissue disease: a clinicopathologic study of 20 cases. Semin Arthritis Rheum 1980;10(1):25–51.

[20] Lash AD, Wittman AL, Quismorio Jr FP. Myocarditis in mixed connective tissue disease: clinical and pathologic study of three cases and review of the literature. Semin Arthritis Rheum 1986; 15(4):288–96.

[21] Lundberg I, Nyman U, Pettersson I, et al. Clinical manifestations and anti-(U1)snRNP antibodies: a prospective study of 29 anti-RNP antibody positive patients. Br J Rheumatol 1992;31(12):811–7.

[22] Bennett RM, O'Connell DJ. The arthritis of mixed connective tissue disease. Ann Rheum Dis 1978;37(5):397–403.

[23] Halla JT, Hardin JG. Clinical features of the arthritis of mixed connective tissue disease. Arthritis Rheum 1978;21(5):497–503.

[24] Ramos-Niembro F, Alarcon-Segovia D, Hernandez-Ortiz J. Articular manifestations of mixed connective tissue disease. Arthritis Rheum 1979;22(1):43–51.

[25] Coppo P, Clauvel JP, Bengoufa D, et al. Inflammatory myositis associated with anti-U1-small nuclear ribonucleoprotein antibodies: a subset of myositis associated with a favourable outcome. Rheumatology (Oxford) 2002;41(9):1040–6.

[26] Lundberg I, Nennesmo I, Hedfors E. A clinical, serological, and histopathological study of myositis patients with and without anti-RNP antibodies. Semin Arthritis Rheum 1992;22(2): 127–38.

[27] Alpert MA, Goldberg SH, Singsen BH, et al. Cardiovascular manifestations of mixed connective tissue disease in adults. Circulation 1983;68:1182–93.

[28] Kasukawa R, Nishimaki T, Takagi T, et al. Pulmonary hypertension in connective tissue disease. Clinical analysis of sixty patients in multi-institutional study. Clin Rheumatol 1990;9(1):56–62.

[29] Alpert MA, Pressly TA, Mukerji V, et al. Acute and long-term effects of nifedipine on pulmonary and systemic hemodynamics in patients with pulmonary hypertension associated with diffuse systemic sclerosis, the CREST syndrome and mixed connective tissue disease. Am J Cardiol 1991;68(17):1687–91.

[30] Rebollar-Gonzalez V, Torre-Delgadillo A, Orea-Tejeda A, et al. Cardiac conduction disturbances in mixed connective tissue disease. Rev Invest Clin 2001;53(4):330–4.

[31] Hammann C, Genton CY, Delabays A, et al. Myocarditis of mixed connective tissue disease: favourable outcome after intravenous pulsed cyclophosphamide. Clin Rheumatol 1999;18(1): 85–7.

[32] Doria A, Ruffatti A, Calligaro A, et al. Antiphospholipid antibodies in mixed connective tissue disease. Clin Rheumatol 1992;11(1):48–50.

[33] Komatireddy GR, Wang GS, Sharp GC, et al. Antiphospholipid antibodies among anti-U1–70 kDa autoantibody positive patients with mixed connective tissue disease. J Rheumatol 1997; 24(2):319–22.

[34] Kitchiner D, Edmonds J, Bruneau C, et al. Mixed connective tissue disease with digital gangrene. Br Med J 1975;1(5952):249–50.

[35] Maddison PJ. Mixed connective tissue disease: overlap syndromes. Baillieres Best Pract Res Clin Rheumatol 2000;14(1):111–24.

[36] Marshall JB, Kretschmar JM, Gerhardt DC, et al. Gastrointestinal manifestations of mixed connective tissue disease. Gastroenterology 1990;98(5 Pt 1):1232–8.

[37] Doria A, Bonavina L, Anselmino M, et al. Esophageal involvement in mixed connective tissue disease. J Rheumatol 1991;18(5):685–90.

[38] Kitridou RC, Akmal M, Turkel SB, et al. Renal involvement in mixed connective tissue disease: a longitudinal clinicopathologic study. Semin Arthritis Rheum 1986;16(2):135–45.

[39] Bodolay E, Bettembuk P, Balogh A, et al. Osteoporosis in mixed connective tissue disease. Clin Rheumatol 2003;22(3):213–7.

RHEUMATIC
DISEASE CLINICS
OF NORTH AMERICA

ELSEVIER
SAUNDERS

Rheum Dis Clin N Am 31 (2005) 549–565

Treatment of Mixed Connective Tissue Disease

Paul Kim, MD*, Jennifer M. Grossman, MD

*Division of Rheumatology, University of California at Los Angeles, Box 951670,
1000 Veteran Avenue, Los Angeles, CA 90095-1670, USA*

The term mixed connective tissue disease (MCTD) was coined by Sharp and colleagues [1] in 1972 to describe a group of patients who had overlapping clinical features of systemic lupus erythematosus (SLE), scleroderma, and polymyositis (PM). MCTD was considered to be distinct because all of these patients exhibited high titers of autoantibodies to a ribonuclease-sensitive component of extractable nuclear antigen [1], later identified as U1 ribonucleoprotein (RNP) [2,3]. Initial descriptions of this syndrome emphasized a good prognosis with an excellent response to corticosteroid therapy and the absence of significant renal or central nervous system involvement [1,4]; however, subsequent studies with longer periods of observations have shown that MCTD is not invariably benign, accompanying organ involvement may be significant, and some clinical manifestations are not responsive to steroids [5–9]. Furthermore, poor prognosis has been associated with pulmonary hypertension, which occurs in certain subsets of patients who have MCTD and causes significant morbidity and mortality [5,9]. Pulmonary hypertension represents the most common disease-related cause of death in MCTD and may be an important target for early aggressive treatment.

Historical perspective on treatment of mixed connective tissue disease

In the initial report by Sharp and colleagues [1], MCTD seemed to be responsive to corticosteroid therapy with a favorable prognosis over a short-term observational period (2 months to 8 years). Of the 25 original patients, 21 who had "major organ involvement" were treated with corticosteroids (usual starting

---

* Corresponding author.
E-mail address: pkim@mednet.ucla.edu (P. Kim).

dosage of prednisone, 1 mg/kg) and 7 also received an alkylating agent. All responded favorably with improvement in myositis, serositis, arthritis, lymphadenopathy, hepatosplenomegaly, fever, anemia, and leukopenia. Some even had improvement in their skin swelling and thickening. More than 70% of treated patients received only one course of high-dose corticosteroids (prednisone, 1 mg/kg) with significant improvement in their clinical manifestations. The remaining 28% required repeated courses for recurrent or persistently active disease. At the end of the follow-up period, all 25 patients were alive and nearly all had a favorable response to steroids; 7 were off therapy, 10 were receiving prednisone at 10 mg or less daily, and only 4 were on prednisone at more than 10 mg/d [1].

Subsequent long-term follow-up studies [5–9], however, have not supported Sharp and colleagues' initial optimistic outlook on MCTD. In particular, extended observations have revealed that not all patients who have MCTD have a benign clinical course and that not all clinical features are steroid responsive. These observations were documented first in the follow-up report of the original 25 patients by Nimelstein and colleagues [8]. In 22 patients who were available for review, inflammatory manifestations (ie, arthritis, serositis, fever, myositis, and skin rash) had improved significantly following corticosteroid treatment, whereas sclerodermatous features (ie, Raynaud's phenomenon [RP], sclerodactyly, esophageal disease, sclerodermatous bowel disease, and chronic pulmonary interstitial disease) persisted and often were unresponsive to therapy. Additionally, 8 patients had died. At least 2 of the deaths could have been attributed to an underlying rheumatic process or a complication related to its treatment. One died of scleroderma-like renal crisis, whereas the other died of respiratory infection while receiving immunosuppression for renal involvement. Although many surviving patients did well and were off therapy or required only low-dose maintenance steroids, overall mortality was high in this group (36%) and sclerodermatous features were persistent and often refractory to treatment.

Several longitudinal studies of patients who have MCTD and anti–U1-RNP antibodies have since been published and confirmed the variable clinical course and prognosis in MCTD; it ranges from benign self-limited disease with little or no steroid requirements to a severe progressive course that is characterized by proliferative vasculopathy with pulmonary hypertension and increased mortality [5–10]. In the most recent longitudinal study of 47 patients who had MCTD who were followed for a mean of 15 years, 17 (36%) were in remission (prednisone <6 mg/d and no cytotoxic drug therapy) following treatment with corticosteroids of varying doses (low, moderate, or high) with (n = 9) or without (n = 8) cyclophosphamide ($\geq$ 50 mg/d); 12 (26%) were improved but still receiving prednisone at less than 20 mg/d; and 18 (38%) responded less favorably to treatment (7 [15%] had persistently active disease, despite aggressive immunosuppression and 11 [23%] had died) [5]. In general, inflammatory manifestations markedly improved with treatment in these patients, whereas sclerodactyly, pulmonary involvement, and nervous system disease tended to persist [5].

Overview of treatment

Despite its original description as being extremely responsive to cortico-steroids with a favorable prognosis [1,4], MCTD is believed to be incurable and seems to have a variable prognosis [5–9]. Some patients may have mild self-limited disease that requires minimal intervention, whereas others may develop severe major organ involvement with life-threatening manifestations that re-quire aggressive treatment. No randomized controlled trials have been performed to help guide therapy in MCTD. Therefore, management of MCTD must be based largely upon the known effectiveness of conventional treatments that are used for similar manifestations in other rheumatic conditions (SLE, scleroderma, and PM) as well as the information that is available from case reports and longitu-dinal experience with several MCTD cohorts over the years. Corticosteroids and cytotoxic agents, most often cyclophosphamide, are the most frequently used immu-nosuppressants, although antimalarials, methotrexate, and vasodilators have been used with varying degrees of success. Given the heterogeneous clinical course of the disease, therapy in MCTD should be individualized for each patient to ad-dress the specific organs involved and the severity of underlying disease activity.

In general, inflammatory manifestations of MCTD that overlap with SLE or PM tend to respond to corticosteroid therapy. These include serositis, skin rash, arthritis, aseptic meningitis, myocarditis, myositis, lymphadenopathy, anemia, and leukopenia. Occasionally, cytotoxic agents may be needed for more extensive organ involvement. In contrast, scleroderma-like features, such as RP, acroscle-rosis, and pulmonary hypertension often are unresponsive to corticosteroid therapy. Peripheral neuropathies, nephrotic syndrome, and severe deforming arthropathy also have been noted to be resistant to therapy. Gastrointestinal manifestations of MCTD frequently overlap with scleroderma and can be managed similarly [11]. A notable exception to this may be the potential benefit of steroid therapy in those who have esophageal involvement in MCTD [12]. Because pulmonary hypertension represents the main cause of death in patients who have MCTD, early diagnosis seems to be important because therapies have shown promise in reducing the morbidity and, perhaps, mortality that are associated with this condition. These include intravenous prostacyclin, trepros-tinil (subcutaneous prostacyclin analog), and bosentan (dual endothelin receptor antagonist), which have demonstrated efficacy in improving exercise capacity, hemodynamics, and clinical symptoms [13–17]. Recommendations for organ-based management for more common problems in MCTD are summarized in Table 1 and are reviewed in greater details in the sections below.

Treatment approach by organ systems

Skin and mucous membranes

Mucocutaneous involvement is common in MCTD. RP is the most common problem and usually occurs early in the course of the disease [1,18,19]. It may

Table 1
Organ-based management recommendations for more common problems in mixed connective tissue disease

Organ-specific problems	Treatment
Constitutional	
Fever	Rule out occult infection/neoplasm. Assess underlying disease activity. Use NSAIDs or steroids (0.25–1.0 mg/kg) for coexistent myositis, serositis, and aseptic meningitis
Fatigue, arthralgias, myalgias	Use NSAIDs, antimalarials, and low-dose steroids (prednisone < 10 mg/d). Assess for fibromyalgia or depression. Treat as indicated.
Skin	
Systemic lupus erythematosus–like rash, photosensitivity	Use preventive measures (avoid sun, use of sunscreens), topical steroids, and antimalarials. *Severe or refractory cases:* systemic steroids, immunosuppression (i.e. azathioprine).
Raynaud's phenomenon	Keep warm, avoid triggers (caffeine, smoking), protect fingers from injury. Use calcium channel blockers (nifedipine, amlodipine) first-line, titrate dose as needed or tolerated. Consider topical nitroglycerin, prazocin, losartan, fluoxetine, or bosentan.
Acute digital ischemia or gangrene	Prostaglandin infusion therapy, digital sympathectomy, or bosentan.
Arthritis	
Mild and nonerosive	Use NSAIDs, antimalarials, low-dose steroids (prednisone ≤ 20 mg/d) for flares
Severe or erosive	Use disease-modifying agents such as methotrexate, unless contraindicated; may consider leflunomide or azathioprine. *Severe deformities:* consider leflunomide or azathioprine, soft tissue release, or joint-fusion surgeries.
Cardiovascular	
Pericarditis	Use NSAIDs or steroids (0.25–1.0 mg/kg). Percutaneous and surgical drainage in rare cases of large effusion with tamponade.
Myocarditis	*Acute moderate-to-severe disease:* trial of high-dose steroids (often pulse, then 1 mg/kg) and cyclophosphamide. Heart failure therapies as needed. Avoid digoxin (predisposes to ventricular arrhythmias).
Pulmonary	
Pleurisy	Use NSAIDs or short-course steroids (0.25–1.0 mg/kg).
Interstial lung disease	Trial of high-dose steroids and cyclophosphamide, azathioprine, or MMF for active alveolitis.
Pulmonary hypertension	Early diagnosis essential for institution of potentially effective therapies. *Mild (PAP 25–35 mmHg) stable:* serial PFTs/echocardiography to monitor any signs of progression.

(continued on next page)

Table 1 (*continued*)

Organ-specific problems	Treatment
	Consider therapy with calcium channel blocker, ACE inhibitor, and/or immunosuppression. *Moderate-to-severe (PAP > 35 mmHg) and progressive:* Referral for right heart catheterization or vasodilator trial. Consider newer vasodilator therapies in addition to anticoagulation (low-dose to INR 1.5–2.0), aggressive immunosuppression, and ACE inhibitors.
Gastrointestinal	
Esophageal reflux or dysphagia	Use proton pump inhibitors, H2 antagonists, and antacids. Life-style modification. Trial of steroids (prednisone 15–30 mg/d) if refractory to conventional therapies. Endoscopic dilatation for severe dysphagia related to strictures and mucosal rings.
Constipation	Increase fiber and fluid intake and exercise. Bowel rest in severe cases (ie, pseudo-obstruction). Use of octreotide?
Muscle	
Myositis	Steroids (0.5–1.0 mg/kg). Consider methotrexate or IVIG.
Renal	
Membranous glomerulonephropathy	*Mild:* no treatment required. *More severe:* trial of steroids (0.25–1.0 mg/kg) and ACE inhibitor. *Nephrotic syndrome:* chlorambucil or cyclophosphamide.
Renal crisis, scleroderma-like	Use ACE inhibitors.
Neuropsychiatric	
Aseptic meningitis	Discontinue NSAIDs (sulindac, ibuprofen associated with hypersensitivity meningitis). Short course of high-dose steroids (1 mg/kg).
Trigeminal neuropathy	Steroids not helpful. Consider antiepileptics, antispasmodics, TCAs, or SSRIs.
Hematologic	
Autoimmune hemolytic anemia, thrombocytopenia	High-dose steroids (1 mg/kg) with taper as tolerated. Use IVIG, danazol or immunosuppression in refractory cases.
TTP	Plasmapheresis and immunosuppression.

Abbreviations: ACE, angiotensin-converting enzyme; INR, international normalized ratio; IVIG, intravenous immune globulin; MCTD, mixed connective tissue disease; MMF, mycophenolate mofetil; NSAIDs, nonsteroidal anti-inflammatory drugs; PAP, pulmonary artery pressure; PFT, pulmonary function test; SSRI, selective serotonin reuptake inhibitor; TCA, tricyclic antidepressant; TNF, tumor necrosis factor; TTP, thrombotic thrombocytopenic purpura.

be associated with digital necrosis in severe cases and represents a major cause of morbidity. Two thirds of patients also develop swollen hands and fingers that leads to a sausage-like appearance of the digits [1]. The skin of the hands may be taut and thick and resemble scleroderma histologically. Other less common manifestations include erythematous eruptions that are similar to SLE, dermatomyositis-like rash, orogenital ulceration, nasal septal perforation, and sicca complex [19–22].

SLE-like skin rash, oral ulcerations, photosensitivity, and occasionally, hand edema have been treated effectively with topical steroids, oral steroids, and/or hydroxychloroquine [1,5,8,19,23]. Sclerodermatous-like skin manifestations often are unresponsive to therapy. RP generally is responsive to conventional vasodilator therapies (ie, calcium channel blockers) in addition to preventive/ nonpharmacologic measures. In some cases, improvement also was noted with immunosuppression (steroids and alkylating agent) [5]. Prostaglandin-infusion therapy was reported to be beneficial in the treatment of severe ischemic digital lesions [24]. Recent reports also have suggested the potential role of bosentan (dual endothelin receptor antagonist) in the treatment of severe RP as well as in the prevention of new digital ulcers in patients who have scleroderma [25,26]. Other novel therapies are discussed in great detail in the article by Wigley and colleagues elsewhere in this issue.

Authors' approach

Lupus-like skin rash and photosensitivity usually can be treated with preventive measures (sun avoidance, daily use of sunscreen lotion), topical steroids, or antimalarials (hydroxychloroquine or in combination with quinacrine). Systemic corticosteroids or other immunosuppressive agents rarely are needed but may be considered in more severe cases. Intravenous immune globulin (IVIG) also may have a role in the treatment of severe, eruptive skin disease that is refractory to other therapies [27]. For RP, initial management should emphasize avoidance of cold temperatures and other triggering factors (caffeine, smoking, sympathomimetic agents), the use of hand and body warming techniques, and protection of fingers from injury. In more severe cases, particularly in the presence of digital ulcerations, vasodilator therapy should be started promptly. Calcium channel blockers (sustained-release nifedipine or amlodipine) remain first-line therapy with the addition of topical nitroglycerin ointment as needed [28]. Other pharmacologic agents which may be useful include prazocin, losartan, fluoxetine, or pentoxifylline. For severe refractory cases with acute ischemic crisis, prostaglandin infusion therapy, digital sympathectomy, or bosentan can be considered [24,26]. Bosentan also may be effective in preventing the development of new digital ulcers [25].

Constitutional

Fever of unknown origin may be the initial presenting manifestation of MCTD [19]. In this setting, it usually was associated with a coexistent serositis, myositis, or aseptic meningitis. After excluding infectious etiology, fever usually resolved following corticosteroid treatment (15–60 mg/d) for disease activity in these specific organ systems [1,19]. Fatigue, arthralgias, and myalgias also are common in MCTD and have been responsive to treatment with nonsteroidal anti-inflammatory drugs (NSAIDs), antimalarials, or low-dose prednisone (< 10 mg/d) [1,7,19].

Authors' approach

For fever that is associated with MCTD, initial evaluation should include a careful search for the presence of occult infection or neoplasm as well as assessment of underlying disease activity. After the former possibilities are excluded, a trial of NSAIDs or corticosteroids (0.25–1.0 mg/kg) should be considered. Therapy can be tailored further for the appropriate treatment of coexistent myositis, serositis, or aseptic meningitis, if identified. Fatigue, arthralgias, and myalgias usually can be controlled with NSAIDs, antimalarials, or low-dose prednisone (< 10 mg/d). The possibility of fibromyalgia or reactive depression always should be considered and addressed appropriately, if present.

Arthritis

Polyarthralgia is an early and common symptom in MCTD. A symmetric polyarthritis that resembles rheumatoid arthritis (RA) occurs in approximately 60% of patients and may be accompanied by joint deformities and characteristic mild erosive changes on radiographs [19,29]. Destructive arthritis, however, including an arthritis mutilans type, also has been described in MCTD [30–32]. Small peritendinous nodules near tendons of forearms and hands have been reported in some patients [33]. Additionally, rheumatoid factor may be positive in up to 70% of patients who have MCTD [1,19,34].

Most patients who have joint symptoms have been treated with NSAIDs, hydroxychloroquine, and/or oral steroids with good response [1,5,7,8,19,23]. Methotrexate has been reported to be useful in patients who have more severe or erosive joint disease, as in RA. Additionally, two case reports were published on the use of anti–tumor necrosis factor (TNF) agents for refractory RA-like polyarthritis in MCTD [35]. Although excellent response for the joint symptoms was observed, both patients developed a lupus-like syndrome that was characterized by systemic illness (fever, malaise, anemia, myalgia/arthralgia), appearance of double-stranded DNA antibodies, and development of hypocomplementemia which resolved following discontinuation of the drug.

Authors' approach

All patients who have arthritis should have baseline radiographs to determine if erosive changes are present. Arthralgias and mild nonerosive arthritis should be treated first with NSAIDs and hydroxychloroquine. Some NSAIDs, particularly sulindac and ibuprofen, have been associated with an increased risk of aseptic meningitis (hypersensitivity-type) in the setting of MCTD and should be used with caution [36,37]. If joint symptoms persist, a trial of low-dose corticosteroids (≤ 10 mg/d) may be helpful. For refractory synovitis or erosive disease, methotrexate should be started as in the management of RA. If methotrexate is contraindicated, other disease-modifying agents, like leflunomide or azathioprine, may be considered. Use of anti-TNF agents is not recommended routinely at this time, and if used, patients should be followed cautiously for the development of a lupus-like syndrome. Surgical interventions, such as soft tissue release operations and selected joint fusions, also may be helpful in patients who have severe hand deformities.

Cardiovascular

Major cardiovascular abnormalities are uncommon in MCTD. Pericarditis is the most common clinical manifestation, occurs in 10% to 30% of patients, and rarely is complicated by pericardial tamponade [1,10,19,38]. The myocardium may be involved with an inflammatory myocarditis or may be damaged secondary to pulmonary hypertension [9,10,38–40]. Electrocardiographic abnormalities occur in 20% of patients and include right ventricular hypertrophy, right atrial enlargement, and interventricular conduction defects [10]. Antimalarials should be avoided in patients who have incomplete heart block because it may predispose to complete heart block [41]. Vasculopathy in MCTD is similar to scleroderma, and is characterized by a bland intimal proliferation and medial hypertrophy that affects small- and medium-sized vessels [39]. Abnormal nailfold capillaroscopy similar to that of scleroderma is common in MCTD and may be associated with pulmonary vascular disease [9,42].

Most patients who had pericarditis were treated with NSAIDs and varying doses of corticosteroids (15–100 mg/d) with good response [1,5,7,8,19,23]. In contrast, patients who had myocarditis tended to relapse with occasional rapid disease progression after initial response to corticosteroids, and often required additional therapies with azathioprine, cyclophosphamide, or IVIG with variable response [39,40,43].

Authors' approach

Typically, pericarditis is mild and usually can be treated with NSAIDs, especially indomethacin. If symptoms persist, corticosteroids (0.25–1.0 mg/kg) can be added. In the rare case of a large effusion with cardiac tamponade, percutaneous or surgical drainage may be necessary. As in SLE, myocarditis can be life-threatening and requires aggressive treatment in severe cases. Therefore, acute presentation of moderate to severe myocarditis should be treated with high-dose steroid therapy (pulse steroids for 3 days followed by 1 mg/kg) with the usual therapy for congestive heart failure, if present. Digoxin should be avoided in this setting given the possible predisposition to ventricular arrhythmias. Cyclophosphamide can be added in more severe refractory cases. IVIG, azathioprine, and mycophenolate mofetil also may be considered.

Pulmonary

Pleuropulmonary involvement is common in MCTD but may be asymptomatic in most cases [9]. The most common clinical manifestations include dyspnea, pleuritic chest pain, and bibasilar rales [9,44]. Radiographic findings include interstitial changes, pleural effusions, pneumonic infiltrates, and pleural thickening. A reduction in carbon monoxide diffusion capacity (DLCO) is the most common abnormality on the pulmonary function test (PFT). Interstitial lung disease (ILD), although usually steroid responsive, may be rapidly progressive in some cases [9,44,45]. Cases of acute interstitial pneumonia and pulmonary hemorrhage have been reported [46–48]. Pulmonary hypertension occurs frequently in MCTD and is the primary disease-associated cause of death [5,9]. It is characterized by a bland intimal proliferation and medial hypertrophy of pulmonary arterioles and may be associated with scleroderma-type capillary changes on nailfold capillaroscopy and the presence of anticardiolipin antibodies [5,9,10,49].

Patients who have pleurisy generally have responded well to treatment with NSAIDs and varying doses of corticosteroids (10–60 mg/d) [1,5,7–9,19,23]. In some patients, pleurisy was self-limited and resolved without treatment. ILD in the context of MCTD has been variably responsive to corticosteroids and immunosuppressive agents, most commonly cyclophosphamide [9,44,50]. Acute inflammatory components were responsive to therapy, whereas sclerodermatous features (ie, pulmonary fibrosis) were not. Pulmonary hypertension in MCTD has been associated with significant morbidity and mortality. Discussion of this important topic is addressed in great detail in the article by Badesch and colleagues elsewhere in this issue. Briefly, recent advances in the management of primary pulmonary hypertension have expanded the treatment options greatly for this potentially devastating complication in MCTD. These include intravenous prostacyclin, treprostinil (subcutaneous prostacyclin analog), sildenafil (PDE5 inhibitor), and bosentan (dual endothelin receptor blocker), all of which were shown to improve exercise capacity, hemodynamics, and clinical symptoms [13–17]. In addition, prolonged immunosuppression with steroids and cyclophosphamide was reported to be helpful in some cases of pulmonary hypertension that were associated with MCTD [9].

Authors' approach

Mild cases of pleurisy usually can be treated with NSAIDs. As with other connective tissue disorders, the possibility of infection or thromboembolic event (ie, pulmonary embolism) also must be excluded. If symptoms persist, a short course of corticosteroids (0.25–1.0 mg/kg) generally is effective. Immunosuppressive agents rarely are indicated for the treatment of pleurisy. For ILD that is associated with MCTD, aggressive immunosuppression should be considered if active alveolitis is suggested by findings on high-resolution CT (ground-glass opacity), bronchoalveolar lavage (neutrophils > 3% or eosinophils > 2%) or PFT (reduced DLCO). Immunosuppressive regimen may consist of high-dose steroids (1 mg/kg or pulse for 3 days if severe) with or without cyclophosphamide (2 mg/kg orally with close monitoring of white blood cell count), azathioprine (target dose 2 mg/kg), or mycophenolate mofetil (2–3 g/d). In regards to pulmonary hypertension, early detection is essential for institution of potentially effective therapies. All patients who have MCTD should undergo screening PFT, echocardiography, and high-resolution CT at the time of diagnosis to look for the presence of pulmonary hypertension. Mild cases (mean pulmonary artery pressure 25–35 mm Hg on echocardiogram) can be followed with serial testing to monitor for any signs of progression. Medical therapy also may be considered at this stage. For moderate to severe cases (mean pulmonary artery pressure > 35 mm Hg on echocardiogram), right heart catheterization with vasodilator trial should be performed. Current therapeutic options for pulmonary hypertension in MCTD include the newer vasodilator therapies (intravenous prostacyclin, treprostinil and bosentan) in addition to the traditional regimen of calcium channel blockers, angiotensin-converting enzyme (ACE) inhibitors, immunosuppression (corticosteroids or cyclophosphamide), and conventional heart failure therapies (anticoagulants, diuretics, cardiac glycosides, and supplemental oxygen).

Gastrointestinal

Gastrointestinal (GI) involvement is common (60%–80%) in MCTD and represents a major feature of overlap with scleroderma [12]. Esophageal manometry is abnormal in up to 85% of patients, changes consist of decreased lower esophageal sphincter pressure, reduced amplitude of peristalsis in distal esophagus, and occasionally, reduced upper sphincter pressure [12]. Often, esophageal dysfunction initially is subclinical with heartburn and dysphagia being the most common symptoms. More diffuse extraesophageal GI involvement, which is similar to that in scleroderma can occur, including malabsorption syndrome and wide-mouthed colonic diverticula [51–53]. Other reported GI manifestations in MCTD include mesenteric vasculitis, colonic perforation, protein-losing enteropathy, chronic active hepatitis, acute pancreatitis, duodenal hemorrhage, pneumatosis intestinalis, hemoperitoneum, hematobilia, secretory diarrhea, and constipation [54–62].

In contrast to scleroderma, esophageal dysfunction was noted to improve following corticosteroid therapy in a longitudinal study of 34 patients who had MCTD; 10 patients who underwent manometry evaluations before and after the initiation of corticosteroid treatment (average dosage, 25 mg/d for a mean duration of 67 weeks) had a statistically significant improvement in lower esophageal pressure and a trend toward improvement in esophageal body peristaltic pressures [12]. Similarly, corticosteroid treatment was associated with improvement in upper esophageal sphincter hypotension and a reduction in the frequency of associated aspiration events in one case report.

Authors' approach

Many of the GI manifestations in MCTD can be managed according to the recommendations for similar disorders in scleroderma [11]. Additionally, a trial of steroid therapy (15–30 mg/d) may be considered in some cases of esophageal dysfunction that are refractory to conventional treatments, that consist of proton-pump inhibitors (PPI), H2 receptor antagonists, antacids, and lifestyle modifications. Esophageal pH monitoring also may be helpful in patients who have persistent reflux symptoms on PPI to determine if high-dose therapy is needed. Severe cases of dysphagia that are related to strictures or mucosal rings may require endoscopic dilatation. Screening for Barrett's esophagus is recommended for long-standing reflux disease.

Constipation is common and should be managed with fluids, fiber, and exercise. Pseudo-obstruction and pneumatosis intestinalis are more severe manifestations and may require hospitalization for bowel rest. Octreotide also may be useful.

Muscle

Myalgias are common in MCTD [1,19]. Frank myositis, however, with significant weakness, electromyographic abnormalities, or muscle enzyme elevations occur less commonly. Inflammatory myopathy that is associated with MCTD is identical clinically and histologically to PM [19]. In most patients, myositis presents acutely in the setting of general disease activity and may be associated with significant fever. Less commonly, patients may present with a more insidious onset, low-grade, persistent myopathy.

Most patients who have acute-onset severe myositis, often with accompanying fever, have been treated with moderate to high doses of corticosteroids (30–100 mg/d) with good response [1,5,7,8,19]. Some reports have suggested a more favorable prognosis for muscle disease in MCTD when compared with PM with less steroid requirements [7,8].

Authors' approach

Myalgias in the absence of myositis usually can be treated with NSAIDs, antimalarials, and/or low-dose prednisone (< 10 mg/d). The possibility of noninflammatory muscle aches from coexistent myofascial syndrome or fibromyalgia should be considered and addressed appropriately, if suspected. In the case of frank myositis, treatment should be started with corticosteroids (0.5–1.0 mg/kg). If muscle enzyme elevations and symptoms do not improve significantly within 1 to 2 months, methotrexate and/or IVIG therapy should be added for optimal management.

Renal

In contrast to the initial description of MCTD, renal involvement seems to be much more prevalent and may occur to some degree in approximately 25% of patients [1,63,64]. Severe renal disease, however, is rare and the presence of anti–U1-RNP antibodies may be protective against the development of diffuse proliferative glomerulonephritis [1,3,34]. Membranous nephropathy is the most common presentation [63,64]. Although this often is asymptomatic, nephrotic syndrome can develop which may respond to high-dose corticosteroid therapy

[64]. Cases of renovascular hypertensive crisis similar to that of the scleroderma kidney also have been reported [65,66].

Authors' approach

Given the variety of histologic manifestations possible, patients who have MCTD and suspected renal involvement (elevated creatinine and/or > 500 mg proteinuria/d) should be considered for kidney biopsy to help characterize the underlying pathology. Mild forms of membranous glomerulonephropathy require no specific treatment. More severe forms with significant proteinuria may be treated with a trial of corticosteroids (0.25–1.0 mg/kg) and ACE inhibitors. Aggressive use of cholesterol-lowering medications (ie, statins) also is important when lipid abnormalities are present. In the case of overt nephrotic syndrome, steroids alone may not be helpful and another immunosuppressive agent, such as cyclophosphamide, mycophenolate mofetil, or chlorambucil, should be considered. In the rare cases of scleroderma-like renal crisis with accelerated hypertension, ACE inhibitors remain the mainstay of treatment. Angiotensin receptor blockers also may be helpful in this setting.

Neuropsychiatric

In accordance with the original description of the disease, severe central nervous system (CNS) involvement is rare in MCTD. Trigeminal neuropathy is the most common CNS manifestation and may be an early clinical feature of MCTD [67]. In contrast to SLE, frank psychosis and convulsions rarely occur in MCTD [1,67]. Headaches are common and most likely are vascular in origin. Some patients occasionally develop an aseptic meningitis-like picture (fever, meningeal irritation, and suggestive cerebrospinal fluid findings), which rarely has been associated with a hypersensitivity-type reaction to NSAIDs, particularly sulindac and ibuprofen [19,36,37]. Isolated cases of cerebral hemorrhage, transverse myelitis, cauda equina syndrome, retinal vasculitis, progressive multifocal leukoencephalopathy, and peripheral neuropathies have been reported [68–77].

Aseptic meningitis generally has been treated with high doses of steroids (30–100 mg/d) with good response [1,19,67]. In many cases, steroids could be tapered rapidly to a reasonable level within 1 to 2 weeks [67]. Trigeminal neuropathy and peripheral neuropathies have been less responsive to therapy. There have been case reports of successful treatment of transverse myelopathy in MCTD with high-dose steroids, azathioprine, or plasmapheresis [78].

Authors' approach

Vascular headaches can be treated with analgesics, aspirin, propranolol, low-dose tricyclic antidepressants, or selective serotonin reuptake inhibitors. Symptomatic use of triptans also may be helpful for more migraine-like headaches. These agents, however, can cause vasospasms, and therefore, should be avoided in patients who have severe RP. Myofascial trigger points, if present, may benefit from therapeutic injections. Aseptic meningitis should be treated with discontinuation of NSAIDs and a short course of high-dose steroids (1 mg/kg) followed by a rapid taper as tolerated. Transverse myelopathy should be treated promptly with high-dose steroids (1 mg/kg), immunosuppressives (azathioprine or cyclophosphamide), or plasmapheresis to prevent permanent damage to the cord.

Hematologic

Nonspecific hematologic and laboratory abnormalities are common in MCTD. Leukopenia, anemia of chronic disease, broad-based hypergammaglobulinemia, and a positive Coomb's test without frank hemolysis have been reported frequently in patients who have MCTD [3,9,19,34]. Less common associations have included thrombocytopenia, thrombotic thrombocytopenic purpura (TTP), and red cell aplasia. Serologically, all patients, by definition, have positive anti–U1-RNP antibodies. Additionally, up to 70% of patients have a positive rheumatoid factor [3,19,34]. Antiphospholipid antibodies also have been reported in MCTD; anticardiolipin antibodies are associated with pulmonary hypertension but not with thrombotic events [5,79].

Anemia and leukopenia in MCTD tend to correlate with disease activity and generally have been noted to improve with therapies that are used for other organ manifestations [1,5,8]. Occasional cases of severe hemolytic anemia, thrombocytopenia, and red cell aplasia have been treated successfully with high-dose steroids [19,80,81]. There have been case reports of TTP associated with MCTD that were treated with high-dose corticosteroids and plasmapheresis with variable response [82,83].

Authors' approach

Mild anemia or leukopenia does not require any specific therapy. Concomitant iron-deficiency should be ruled out and managed appropriately, if present. Moderate to severe autoimmune hemolytic anemia or thrombocytopenia should be treated with high-dose steroids (1 mg/kg) with subsequent taper as tolerated. As in SLE, steroid-resistant cases may be treated with IVIG, danazol, splenectomy, or other immunosuppressive agents. TTP should be treated with plasmapheresis in addition to immunosuppression.

Summary

MCTD is believed to be incurable and seems to have a variable prognosis. Some patients have a mild self-limited disease, whereas others develop major organ involvement that requires aggressive treatment. Because no controlled clinical trials have been performed to guide therapy in MCTD, treatment strategies must rely largely upon the conventional therapies that are used for similar problems in other rheumatic conditions (SLE, scleroderma, and PM), as well as the experience that is available from case reports and longitudinal cohort studies over the years. Given the heterogeneous clinical course of MCTD, therapy should be individualized for each patient to address the specific organ involved and the severity of underlying disease activity. Corticosteroids, antimalarials, methotrexate, cytotoxics (most often cyclophosphamide), and vasodilators have been used with varying degrees of success. In general, inflammatory manifestations that overlap with SLE or PM tend to be responsive to therapy, whereas sclerodermatous features (particularly RP, acrosclerosis, and pulmonary hypertension) often are unresponsive to therapy. Because pulmonary hypertension represents the main cause of death in patients who have MCTD, early diagnosis seems to be important with institution of potentially effective therapies which may reduce the morbidity, and perhaps, the mortality that are associated with this condition. These include intravenous prostacyclin, treprostinil, sildenafil, and bosentan which have all demonstrated efficacy in improving exercise capacity, hemodynamics, and clinical symptoms.

References

[1] Sharp GC, Irvin WS, Tan EM, et al. Mixed connective tissue disease–an apparently distinct rheumatic disease syndrome associated with a specific antibody to an extractable nuclear antigen (ENA). Am J Med 1972;52(2):148–59.
[2] Lerner MR, Steitz JA. Antibodies to small nuclear RNAs complexed with proteins are produced by patients with systemic lupus erythematosus. Proc Natl Acad Sci USA 1979;76(11):5495–9.
[3] Sharp GC, Irvin WS, May CM, et al. Association of antibodies to ribonucleoprotein and Sm antigens with mixed connective-tissue disease, systematic lupus erythematosus and other rheumatic diseases. N Engl J Med 1976;295(21):1149–54.
[4] Minkin W, Rabhan N. Mixed connective tissue disease. Arch Dermatol 1976;112(11):1535–8.
[5] Burdt MA, Hoffman RW, Deutscher SL, et al. Long-term outcome in mixed connective tissue disease: longitudinal clinical and serologic findings. Arthritis Rheum 1999;42(5):899–909.
[6] Lazaro MA, Maldonado Cocco JA, Catoggio LJ, et al. Clinical and serologic characteristics of patients with overlap syndrome: is mixed connective tissue disease a distinct clinical entity? Medicine (Baltimore) 1989;68(1):58–65.
[7] Lundberg I, Hedfors E. Clinical course of patients with anti-RNP antibodies. A prospective study of 32 patients. J Rheumatol 1991;18(10):1511–9.
[8] Nimelstein SH, Brody S, McShane D, et al. Mixed connective tissue disease: a subsequent evaluation of the original 25 patients. Medicine (Baltimore) 1980;59(4):239–48.
[9] Sullivan WD, Hurst DJ, Harmon CE, et al. A prospective evaluation emphasizing pulmonary involvement in patients with mixed connective tissue disease. Medicine (Baltimore) 1984;63(2):92–107.
[10] Alpert MA, Goldberg SH, Singsen BH, et al. Cardiovascular manifestations of mixed connective tissue disease in adults. Circulation 1983;68(6):1182–93.
[11] Sjogren RW. Gastrointestinal motility disorders in scleroderma. Arthritis Rheum 1994;37(9):1265–82.
[12] Marshall JB, Kretschmar JM, Gerhardt DC, et al. Gastrointestinal manifestations of mixed connective tissue disease. Gastroenterology 1990;98(5 Pt 1):1232–8.
[13] Badesch DB, Tapson VF, McGoon MD, et al. Continuous intravenous epoprostenol for pulmonary hypertension due to the scleroderma spectrum of disease. A randomized, controlled trial. Ann Intern Med 2000;132(6):425–34.
[14] Channick RN, Simonneau G, Sitbon O, et al. Effects of the dual endothelin-receptor antagonist bosentan in patients with pulmonary hypertension: a randomised placebo-controlled study. Lancet 2001;358(9288):1119–23.

[15] Oudiz RJ, Schilz RJ, Barst RJ, et al. Treprostinil, a prostacyclin analogue, in pulmonary arterial hypertension associated with connective tissue disease. Chest 2004;126(2):420–7.

[16] Rubin LJ, Badesch DB, Barst RJ, et al. Bosentan therapy for pulmonary arterial hypertension. N Engl J Med 2002;346(12):896–903.

[17] Simonneau G, Barst RJ, Galie N, et al. Continuous subcutaneous infusion of treprostinil, a prostacyclin analogue, in patients with pulmonary arterial hypertension: a double-blind, randomized, placebo-controlled trial. Am J Respir Crit Care Med 2002;165(6):800–4.

[18] Arcon-Segovia D. Mixed connective tissue disease and overlap syndromes. Clin Dermatol 1994;12(2):309–16.

[19] Bennett RM, O'Connell DJ. Mixed connective tissue disease: a clinicopathologic study of 20 cases. Semin Arthritis Rheum 1980;10(1):25–51.

[20] Hamza M. Orogenital ulcerations in mixed connective tissue disease. J Rheumatol 1985;12(3): 643–4.

[21] Konttinen YT, Tuominen TS, Piirainen HI, et al. Signs and symptoms in the masticatory system in ten patients with mixed connective tissue disease. Scand J Rheumatol 1990;19(5): 363–73.

[22] Willkens RF, Roth GJ, Novak A, et al. Perforation of nasal septum in rheumatic diseases. Arthritis Rheum 1976;19(1):119–21.

[23] Bodolay E, Csiki Z, Szekanecz Z, et al. Five-year follow-up of 665 Hungarian patients with undifferentiated connective tissue disease (UCTD). Clin Exp Rheumatol 2003;21(3):313–20.

[24] Cohen LE, Faske I, Fenske NA, et al. Prostaglandin infusion therapy for intermittent digital ischemia in a patient with mixed connective tissue disease. Case report and review of the literature. J Am Acad Dermatol 1989;20(5 Pt 2):893–7.

[25] Korn JH, Mayes M, Matucci CM, et al. Digital ulcers in systemic sclerosis: prevention by treatment with bosentan, an oral endothelin receptor antagonist. Arthritis Rheum 2004;50(12): 3985–93.

[26] Ramos-Casals M, Brito-Zeron P, Nardi N, et al. Successful treatment of severe Raynaud's phenomenon with bosentan in four patients with systemic sclerosis. Rheumatology (Oxford) 2004;43(11):1454–6.

[27] Ulmer A, Kotter I, Pfaff A, et al. Efficacy of pulsed intravenous immunoglobulin therapy in mixed connective tissue disease. J Am Acad Dermatol 2002;46(1):123–7.

[28] Wigley FM. Clinical practice. Raynaud's Phenomenon. N Engl J Med 2002;347(13):1001–8.

[29] O'Connell DJ, Bennett RM. Mixed connective tissue disease–clinical and radiological aspects of 20 cases. Br J Radiol 1977;50(597):620–5.

[30] Bennett RM, O'Connell DJ. The arthritis of mixed connective tissue disease. Ann Rheum Dis 1978;37(5):397–403.

[31] Halla JT, Hardin JG. Clinical features of the arthritis of mixed connective tissue disease. Arthritis Rheum 1978;21(5):497–503.

[32] Ramos-Niembro F, Arcon-Segovia D, Hernandez-Ortiz J. Articular manifestations of mixed connective tissue disease. Arthritis Rheum 1979;22(1):43–51.

[33] Babini SM, Maldonado-Cocco JA, Barcelo HA, et al. Peritendinous nodules in overlap syndrome. J Rheumatol 1985;12(1):160–4.

[34] Lemmer JP, Curry NH, Mallory JH, et al. Clinical characteristics and course in patients with high titer anti-RNP antibodies. J Rheumatol 1982;9(4):536–42.

[35] Christopher-Stine L, Wigley F. Tumor necrosis factor-alpha antagonists induce lupus-like syndrome in patients with scleroderma overlap/mixed connective tissue disease. J Rheumatol 2003; 30(12):2725–7.

[36] Hoffman M, Gray RG. Ibuprofen-induced meningitis in mixed connective tissue disease. Clin Rheumatol 1982;1(2):128–30.

[37] Yasuda Y, Akiguchi I, Kameyama M. Sulindac-induced aseptic meningitis in mixed connective tissue disease. Clin Neurol Neurosurg 1989;91(3):257–60.

[38] Nunoda S, Mifune J, Ono S, et al. An adult case of mixed connective tissue disease associated with perimyocarditis and massive pericardial effusion. Jpn Heart J 1986;27(1):129–35.

[39] Lash AD, Wittman AL, Quismorio Jr FP. Myocarditis in mixed connective tissue disease: clinical and pathologic study of three cases and review of the literature. Semin Arthritis Rheum 1986;15(4):288–96.

[40] Whitlow PL, Gilliam JN, Chubick A, et al. Myocarditis in mixed connective tissue disease. Association of myocarditis with antibody to nuclear ribonucleoprotein. Arthritis Rheum 1980; 23(7):808–15.

[41] Black C, Isenberg DA. Mixed connective tissue disease–goodbye to all that. Br J Rheumatol 1992;31(10):695–700.

[42] Peller JS, Gabor GT, Porter JM, et al. Angiographic findings in mixed connective tissue disease. Correlation with fingernail capillary photomicroscopy and digital photoplethysmography findings. Arthritis Rheum 1985;28(7):768–74.

[43] Hammann C, Genton CY, Delabays A, et al. Myocarditis of mixed connective tissue disease: favourable outcome after intravenous pulsed cyclophosphamide. Clin Rheumatol 1999;18(1): 85–7.

[44] Prakash UB, Luthra HS, Divertie MB. Intrathoracic manifestations in mixed connective tissue disease. Mayo Clin Proc 1985;60(12):813–21.

[45] Wiener-Kronish JP, Solinger AM, Warnock ML, et al. Severe pulmonary involvement in mixed connective tissue disease. Am Rev Respir Dis 1981;124(4):499–503.

[46] Germain MJ, Davidman M. Pulmonary hemorrhage and acute renal failure in a patient with mixed connective tissue disease. Am J Kidney Dis 1984;3(6):420–4.

[47] Sanchez-Guerrero J, Cesarman G, Arcon-Segovia D. Massive pulmonary hemorrhage in mixed connective tissue diseases. J Rheumatol 1989;16(8):1132–4.

[48] Suzuki M, Shimizu K, Sakamoto K, et al. [Interstitial pneumonia associated with mixed connective tissue disease–marked improvement with azathioprine]. Nihon Kyobu Shikkan Gakkai Zasshi 1996;34(1):101–5.

[49] Nishimaki T, Aotsuka S, Kondo H, et al. Immunological analysis of pulmonary hypertension in connective tissue diseases. J Rheumatol 1999;26(11):2357–62.

[50] Prakash UB. Respiratory complications in mixed connective tissue disease. Clin Chest Med 1998;19(4):733–46.

[51] Lynn JT, Gossen G, Miller A, et al. Pneumatosis intestinalis in mixed connective tissue disease: two case reports and literature review. Arthritis Rheum 1984;27(10):1186–9.

[52] Norman DA, Fleischmann RM. Gastrointestinal systemic sclerosis in serologic mixed connective tissue disease. Arthritis Rheum 1978;21(7):811–9.

[53] Samach M, Brandt LJ, Bernstein LH. Spontaneous pneumoperitoneum with Pneumatosis cystoides intestinalis in a patient with mixed connective tissue disease. Am J Gastroenterol 1978;69(4):494–500.

[54] Cooke CL, Lurie HI. Case report: fatal gastrointestinal hemorrhage in mixed connective tissue disease. Arthritis Rheum 1977;20(7):1421–7.

[55] Haas C, Fadlallah JP, Lowenstein W, et al. [Apparently primary pulmonary arterial hypertension complicating systemic diseases. Epidemiological survey and review of the literature]. Ann Med Interne (Paris) 1992;143(4):261–8.

[56] Hameenkorpi R, Hakala M, Ruuska P, et al. Thyroid disorder in patients with mixed connective tissue disease. J Rheumatol 1993;20(3):602–3.

[57] Kuipers EJ, van Leeuwen MA, Nikkels PG, et al. Hemobilia due to vasculitis of the gall bladder in a patient with mixed connective tissue disease. J Rheumatol 1991;18(4):617–8.

[58] Nishimaki T, Aotsuka S, Kunieda T, et al. [Preliminary criteria for the diagnosis of pulmonary hypertension in mixed connective tissue disease]. Ryumachi 1991;31(2):159–66.

[59] Pun YL, Russell DM, Taggart GJ, et al. Pneumatosis intestinalis and pneumoperitoneum complicating mixed connective tissue disease. Br J Rheumatol 1991;30(2):146–9.

[60] Tanimoto K. [Overlapping syndrome]. Nippon Rinsho 1992;50(3):625–8.

[61] Terren P. Protein-losing enteropathy and mixed connective-tissue disease. Med J Aust 1988; 149(10):558–9.

[62] Thiele DL, Krejs GJ. Secretory diarrhea in mixed connective tissue disease. Am J Gastroenterol 1985;80(2):107–10.

[63] Bennett RM, Spargo BH. Immune complex nephropathy in mixed connective tissue disease. Am J Med 1977;63(4):534–41.
[64] Kitridou RC, Akmal M, Turkel SB, et al. Renal involvement in mixed connective tissue disease: a longitudinal clinicopathologic study. Semin Arthritis Rheum 1986;16(2):135–45.
[65] Crapper RM, Dowling JP, Mackay IR, et al. Acute scleroderma in stable mixed connective tissue disease: treatment by plasmapheresis. Aust N Z J Med 1987;17(3):327–9.
[66] Miyata M, Kida S, Kanno T, et al. Pulmonary hypertension in MCTD: report of two cases with anticardiolipin antibody. Clin Rheumatol 1992;11(2):195–201.
[67] Bennett RM, Bong DM, Spargo BH. Neuropsychiatric problems in mixed connective tissue disease. Am J Med 1978;65(6):955–62.
[68] Alpert MA, Pressly TA, Mukerji V, et al. Acute and long-term effects of nifedipine on pulmonary and systemic hemodynamics in patients with pulmonary hypertension associated with diffuse systemic sclerosis, the CREST syndrome and mixed connective tissue disease. Am J Cardiol 1991;68(17):1687–91.
[69] Doria A, Ruffatti A, Calligaro A, et al. Antiphospholipid antibodies in mixed connective tissue disease. Clin Rheumatol 1992;11(1):48–50.
[70] Graf WD, Milstein JM, Sherry DD. Stroke and mixed connective tissue disease. J Child Neurol 1993;8(3):256–9.
[71] Kappes J, Bennett RM. Cauda equina syndrome in a patient with high titer anti-RNP antibodies. Arthritis Rheum 1982;25(3):349–52.
[72] Katada E, Ojika K, Uemura M, et al. Mixed connective tissue disease associated with acute polyradiculoneuropathy. Intern Med 1997;36(2):118–24.
[73] Kraus A, Cervantes G, Barojas E, et al. Retinal vasculitis in mixed connective tissue disease. A fluoroangiographic study. J Rheumatol 1985;12(6):1122–4.
[74] Kuwana M, Kaburaki J, Okano Y, et al. Clinical and prognostic associations based on serum antinuclear antibodies in Japanese patients with systemic sclerosis. Arthritis Rheum 1994;37(1):75–83.
[75] Martyn JB, Wong MJ, Huang SH. Pulmonary and neuromuscular complications of mixed connective tissue disease: a report and review of the literature. J Rheumatol 1988;15(4):703–5.
[76] Pedersen C, Bonen H, Boesen F. Transverse myelitis in mixed connective tissue disease. Clin Rheumatol 1987;6(2):290–2.
[77] Sato M, Yanagisawa K, Matsubara N, et al. [Mixed connective tissue disease–various neuro-muscular complications prior to the elevation of antibody to RNP]. Rinsho Shinkeigaku 1991; 31(10):1143–6.
[78] Mok CC, Lau CS. Transverse myelopathy complicating mixed connective tissue disease. Clin Neurol Neurosurg 1995;97(3):259–60.
[79] Hoffman RW, Greidinger EL. Mixed connective tissue disease. Curr Opin Rheumatol 2000; 12(5):386–90.
[80] Julkunen H, Jantti J, Pettersson T. Pure red cell aplasia in mixed connective tissue disease. J Rheumatol 1989;16(10):1385–6.
[81] Segond P, Yeni P, Jacquot JM, et al. Severe autoimmune anemia and thrombopenia in mixed connective tissue disease. Arthritis Rheum 1978;21(8):995–7.
[82] Kato A, Suzuki Y, Fujigaki Y, et al. Thrombotic thrombocytopenic purpura associated with mixed connective tissue disease. Rheumatol Int 2002;22(3):122–5.
[83] ter Borg EJ, Houtman PM, Kallenberg CG, et al. Thrombocytopenia and hemolytic anemia in a patient with mixed connective tissue disease due to thrombotic thrombocytopenic purpura. J Rheumatol 1988;15(7):1174–7.

ELSEVIER
SAUNDERS

RHEUMATIC
DISEASE CLINICS
OF NORTH AMERICA

Rheum Dis Clin N Am 31 (2005) 567–574

Index

Note: Page numbers of article titles are in **boldface** type.

A

Alarcon-Segovia criteria, for mixed connective tissue disease, 422–423, 509–510

Alveolar hemorrhage, in mixed connective tissue disease, 460–461

Amlodipine, for mixed connective tissue disease, in pediatric patients, 494

Amyloidosis, of kidney, in mixed connective tissue disease, 527

Anemia, in mixed connective tissue disease hemolytic, 528, 553, 561
of chronic disease, 561

Ankylosing spondylitis, in mixed connective tissue disease, 521

Antibody(ies)
in mixed connective tissue disease, 416–417, 429–432, 493
in pediatric patients, 493
in Raynaud's phenomenon, 467–469, 471–472
induction of, 442–443
model for, 445–447
myositis and, 513
prognosis and, 443–445, 536–537
timing of response of, 440–441
types of, 438–440
in scleroderma, 468–469
in systemic lupus erythematosus, 469

Anticardiolipin antibodies, in mixed connective tissue disease, 431, 529, 542

Anticoagulants
for pulmonary hypertension, in connective tissue disease, 455
for Raynaud's phenomenon, in mixed connective tissue disease, 475

Antioxidants, for Raynaud's phenomenon, in mixed connective tissue disease, 475

Antiphospholipid syndrome, in mixed connective tissue disease, 528–529, 542

Antiplatelet therapy, for Raynaud's phenomenon, in mixed connective tissue disease, 475

Arthralgia, in mixed connective tissue disease, 413, 520
in pediatric patients, 487–491
prognosis and, 540–541
treatment of, 552, 555

Arthritis, in mixed connective tissue disease, 413, 423–424, 520–521
in pediatric patients, 487–491
prognosis and, 540–541
rheumatoid, 413–414, 427, 429
treatment of, 552, 555

Arthritis mutilans, in mixed connective tissue disease, 521, 555

Aseptic meningitis, in mixed connective tissue disease, 553, 560

Aspirin, for Raynaud's phenomenon, in mixed connective tissue disease, 475

Atrioventricular block, in mixed connective tissue disease, 528

Autoantibodies. *See* specific antibodies.

Autoimmune hepatitis, in mixed connective tissue disease, 523

Autonomic dysfunction, cardiac, in mixed connective tissue disease, 528

Avascular necrosis, in mixed connective tissue disease, 520, 540

Azathioprine, for mixed connective tissue disease
in pediatric patients, 494
in pulmonary hypertension, 557

B

B lymphocytes, in mixed connective tissue disease, 439, 442–443

Changing Your Address?

Make sure your subscription changes too! When you notify us of your new address, you can help make our job easier by including an exact copy of your Clinics label number with your old address (see illustration below.) This number identifies you to our computer system and will speed the processing of your address change. Please be sure this label number accompanies your old address and your corrected address—you can send an old Clinics label with your number on it or just copy it exactly and send it to the address listed below.

We appreciate your help in our attempt to give you continuous coverage. Thank you.

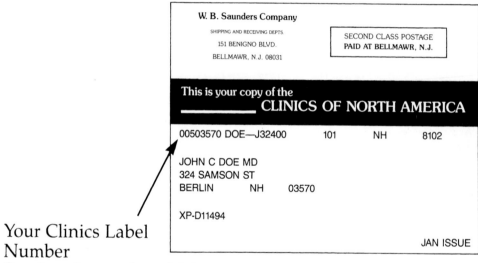

W. B. Saunders Company

SHIPPING AND RECEIVING DEPTS.
151 BENIGNO BLVD.
BELLMAWR, N.J. 08031

SECOND CLASS POSTAGE
PAID AT BELLMAWR, N.J.

This is your copy of the
_____ CLINICS OF NORTH AMERICA

00503570 DOE—J32400   101   NH   8102

JOHN C DOE MD
324 SAMSON ST
BERLIN   NH   03570

XP-D11494

JAN ISSUE

Your Clinics Label Number
Copy it exactly or send your label along with your address to:
W.B. Saunders Company, Customer Service
Orlando, FL 32887-4800
Call Toll Free 1-800-654-2452

Please allow four to six weeks for delivery of new subscriptions and for processing address changes.